M000222189

Anxiety: Panicking about Panic

A powerful, self-help guide
for those suffering from an
Anxiety or Panic Disorder

———

Joshua Fletcher

Anxiety: Panicking about Panic. A powerful, self-help guide for those
suffering from an Anxiety and Panic Disorder
Copyright © 2014 by Joshua Fletcher

All rights reserved.
No part of this book may be reproduced or transmitted in any form or by
any means without written permission from the author.
Second edition 2019. First published 2014.
ISBN: 978-1500117924

Dedication

I dedicate this book to Harry. Thank you for your inspiration during the happiest and darkest of times.

Acknowledgements

I would like to acknowledge the input of many anxiety sufferers from around the world who have shared their stories and experiences through various blogs and forums. These experiences, whether positive or negative, have contributed towards my understanding of the condition and have helped me to write this book.

I would also like to thank Hannah for helping me to edit this book and supporting me through some difficult and challenging times.

Contents

Introduction   **1**

The Symptoms of an Anxiety and Panic problem   **4**

PART 1

1.1 Do I have an anxiety problem?   8

    Anxiety Assumptions   10

    I'm handing out labels and pills. Who wants some?   20

1.2 Why am I panicking and where did this come from?   24

    The Loop of Peaking Anxiety   29

    Why does an anxiety problem start?   33

1.3 Anxiety is Adrenaline and a Sensitive Nervous System   34

    Panic Attacks   38

    Rationality and Worst Case Scenarios   42

PART 2

Anxiety Symptoms Explained   47

PART 3

3.1 It's Just Anxiety   77

Stop trying to work your feelings out!   78

Lose the *'What If?'* because it's just anxiety.   83

It really is 'just anxiety'   87

There's nothing 'wrong' with you   89

The Power of Thought   91

Anxiety should not be feared   94

3.2 Change the bad habits. Re-wire your brain.   95

Stop over-thinking and 'Body checking'   95

Do what you'd usually do, or try something new!   98

Change your reaction and you'll change the anxiety   100

Give yourself something to look forward to   102

Don't associate feeling anxious to future events   104

Stop researching your symptoms on the internet!   106

If you're looking for something then you'll find it   109

3.3 Helpful Anxiety Advice   111

Score your anxiety levels   112

Lose the Emotional Crutches   113

Keep Fit, Eat Healthy   115

Cut down on caffeine and alcohol   119

Patience and discipline   121

The Do's and Do Not's when approaching anxiety   122

My Story   124

PART 4

Emergency Panic Attack Help Page   131

By the Same Author   132

Introduction

HELLO AND THANK YOU for purchasing this book. My name is Josh and for years I suffered with anxiety and unexplainable panic. In April 2012, after confidently stating that I was free from the clutches of excessive anxiety, I decided to write this self-help book for similar people who are struggling with anxiety, worry, panic attacks and the constant overwhelming feeling of fear and dread. This book is strongly tailored towards those who are suffering from a panic disorder or a debilitating anxiety condition.

If you struggle with anxiety and panic, or are perhaps suffering at this very moment, then fear not as this book has been purposely constructed to quickly put your mind at ease. I know that reading or focusing on anything can be difficult when feeling panicky or 'on edge' but stick with me on this one and I assure you that this book has the tools to help you alleviate your current fears. No matter how long you've been suffering for – weeks, months or even years – an anxiety and panic problem can be fixed.

Anxiety, panic and irrational thoughts are debilitating and scary, leading us into depressive states because we believe that we do not function properly as valued human beings with them seemingly ever present. However, just by opening this book, you have given clear evidence that you're striving to do something about this ongoing problem, which in itself is an incredibly brave thing to do. It's also proof that you're not going 'insane' – a common symptom/assumption that many people seem to conclude when battling anxiety – because you've acknowledged something isn't right and by picking up this book you've made a rational, conscious choice to do something about it.

I've written this book as an 'easy to access', self-help guide for those whose lives have been severely affected by panic and the symptoms of anxiety. It has been written from a perspective that takes into regard my own battle with anxiety, as well as using knowledge that has been built up through observations and working with other sufferers.

This book begins with a comprehensive list of symptoms that relate to anxiety, although it primarily addresses anxiety's main symptoms which consist of unexplainable panic, panic attacks, derealisation, hypochondria, continuous fear and hypersensitivity. I believe that these are the root cause of all of the other physical problems that can arise with anxiety, such as heart palpitations, chest pains, headaches, insomnia, dizziness etc.

This book is then split into four main parts: the first part covers the basics of anxiety, panic and what's happening within our minds and bodies when we find ourselves panicking. It's probable you'll find that reading this part of the book imparts a strong form of relief, as it provides an essential tool needed for the recovery process – an understanding of what's actually going on.

Part two is a detailed list of the symptoms that can occur with anxiety. It is set out using a *'What?'* and *'Why?'* format to simplify and explain why such symptoms occur.

Part three offers further information and practical advice to keep anxiety and panic at bay and part four is a short 'emergency relief' section written for those who are experiencing a panic attack.

So, let us begin. Give this book a chance and I'm sure it will help to put your mind at ease.

Worry never robs tomorrow of its sorrow,
it only saps today of its joy

Leo Buscaglia

The symptoms of an anxiety and panic problem

Psychological symptoms:

- **Excessive Worry**
- **Panic Attacks**
- **Derealisation** (feeling lucid and detached from surroundings)
- **Depersonalisation** (feeling detached from persona/personality)
- **Feeling apprehensive**
- **Hypochondria** (The fear that you're seriously ill)
- **The fear of a panic attack**
- **Body checking** (Looking for illness)
- **Repetitive & looping thoughts**
- **Feeling terrified**
- **Obsessive thoughts**
- **Inability to relax**
- **Difficulty completing tasks**
- **Feeling hopeless and depressed**
- **Overactive imagination**
- **Agoraphobia** (fear of going outside)

- **Fear of other people's opinions**
- **Fear of embarrassment**
- **Fear that you're developing a psychological illness**
- **Self-Analysing** (checking the body for signs that something is wrong)
- **Negative thoughts of isolation**
- **Deep level of focus about personal 'identity'**
- **Loss of appetite**
- **Big increase in appetite**
- **Loss of libido**
- **Loss of interest in work**
- **Loss of interest doing things that were once enjoyable**
- **Depressive thoughts**
- **Dwelling on thoughts**
- **Constantly trying to work out how to feel 'normal' again**
- **Constantly feeling tired**
- **Dampened sense of humor**
- **Inability to focus**

Physical symptoms:

+ **Heart palpitations** (short bursts of a rapid heartbeat)
+ **Headaches** – constant or recurring
+ **Light headedness**
+ **Exhaustion**
+ **Constant lethargy**
+ **Irregular bowel movements**
+ **Chest pains** (ache)
+ **Chest pains** (sharp stabbing)
+ **Bloating**
+ **Tickling/fluttering sensation in chest and esophagus**
+ **Nausea**
+ **Constant pacing**
+ **Dizziness**
+ **Perspiration** (sweating frequently)
+ **Tinnitus** (ringing ears)
+ **Stomach cramps**
+ **Eye floaters** (particle-like objects that 'float' in front of vision)
+ **Symptoms of Irritable Bowel Syndrome**
+ **Rib pains**
+ **Rib discomfort** (feeling pressure under ribs)
+ **Stomach grumbling**

- Dry mouth
- Feeling tired after eating
- Abdominal pains
- Shooting pains in back and abdomen
- Neck ache and pains
- Ache behind eyes
- Erectile dysfunction
- Jaw ache and tenderness

PART 1

1.1 Do I have an anxiety problem?

YOU'RE READING THIS BOOK, albeit through probable desperation, because you've acknowledged the fact that something isn't quite right with your mind and body. Perhaps you don't feel like the way that you 'used to', and that your days are often dictated by odd feelings of apprehension and worry. It's also likely that you've often found yourself being struck with bouts of unexplainable panic, which can often trigger a chain of events where you may ultimately begin to panic about the state of panicking itself.

On top of anxious thoughts and panic attacks, maybe you're experiencing the feelings of constant worry, states of derealization (detachment from self and surroundings), an inability to relax, strange bodily changes and depression. Believe it or not, these are all common symptoms of an unbelievably non-complex anxiety condition. Anxiety actually has an overabundance of symptoms, some of which you may have stumbled across at the start of this book. These symptoms, which range from the obvious to the obscure, are all linked to anxiety in some way.

I suggest that you take a look at the comprehensive list and see which of the symptoms can be applied to you and your current state. A lot of these symptoms crop up almost exclusively alongside an ongoing anxiety condition and have direct links to suffering from an anxiety or panic disorder.

Anxiety comes with a lot of baggage and to the uneducated victim it can be a confusing and frightening condition. After my first run-in with anxiety, it didn't take long for me to start foraging desperately for an answer to explain how and why I felt the way I did – a decision which saw my anxiety worsen before it got better. I will explain this in greater depth later on.

'Anxiety' is a word/topic that floats around society and dips in and out of conversation as frequently as talking about the weather. Take these for example: *"I'm anxious about my upcoming interview"*, *"My partner's absence is giving me anxiety"*, *"I can't wait until this is over so I can relax"*, *"This is nail-biting stuff!"* are all common examples of phrases that occur in conversation to describe the way a person is feeling when fearing a possible outcome.

This type of anxiety doesn't seem to be questioned because throughout our lives we have concluded that this type of anxiety is normal. It is *normal* to fear an exam result, the dentist, an operation, public speaking, what the boss will say etc. However, when worrying thoughts and anxious behaviours become a daily constant - for reasons beyond our comprehension - we start to acknowledge and admit to ourselves that something isn't quite right.

The classic and most common sign of an anxiety problem is when we find that our days are mostly being dictated by feelings of intense and unexplainable fear, and that we may begin to perceive everything around us as different and somewhat 'detached'. Further to this, panic may have crept into our lives, which can act as a focus point towards which we direct our worries. This fear can easily lead us to questioning things such as our health, our perception of reality and believing in the most unlikely of worst-case scenarios.

Below are some of the common assumptions that the standard anxiety victim can often relate to:

Anxiety Assumptions

- I feel terrified for no logical reason.

- I haven't felt normal for a long time, something must be wrong.

- Why am I scared to do 'normal' things?

- A psychological condition must be the cause of this change.

- I must have a serious health problem: i.e. heart failure, cancer.

- My brain/mind does not work like those around me.

- I don't think this is ever going to go away. I can't handle it.

- No one else fully understands what I'm going through.

- Why do I feel like I'm about to die?

Furthermore, it is important that we look at some of the most common *physical* symptoms that signal an anxiety problem. The symptoms section at the start of this book supplies a comprehensive list of symptoms that have all been linked to anxiety; below are some I have found to be the most common:

The most common physical symptoms

- **Heart** - Palpitations, chest flutters, 'skipping a beat', heart pounding, hyperawareness of heart beat.

- **Abdominal Pains** - Chest pains and tightness, stomach pains and cramping.

- **Derealisation** - sense of unreality, an illusory detachment from surroundings, shut down of peripheral vision, difficulty focusing.

- **Head** - Constant and prolonged headaches, light headedness, dizziness, vertigo, tinnitus, sensitivity to light, eye floaters.

- **Energy** - Tiredness, lethargy, 'heavy head', exhaustion.

- **Pain** - Unfamiliar aches and pains, cramps, rib pain, muscle tension pain, dental pain.

- **I.B.S** - Indigestion, constipation, acid reflux, trapped wind, diarrhoea, gut and intestinal pains.

If you feel that you can relate to any of the listed anxiety assumptions, and to several of the symptoms listed here and at the start of this book, then it would be a pretty safe bet to assume that you have an anxiety problem.

Fear not as an anxiety problem isn't at all dangerous; it cannot permanently harm you and is something that's easily fixable when fully understood. What has happened - putting it in the most basic of terms - is that your body has arrived at a state of chemical imbalance as a result of trying to deal with high amounts stress and operating using a poor mental routine. In other words, unexplainable anxiety is your body's way of telling you that it has simply had enough and something has to change.

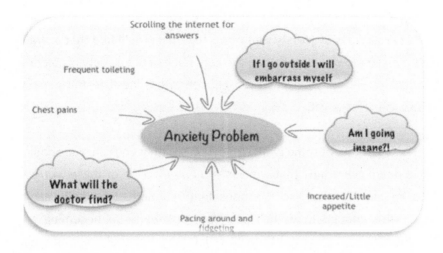

Let's take a look at these anxiety maps that represent some common situations relating to anxiety. I highly recommend making your own as it's a healthy, cathartic way of putting worries on paper. It also helps to clarify and organise problems into one accessible picture.

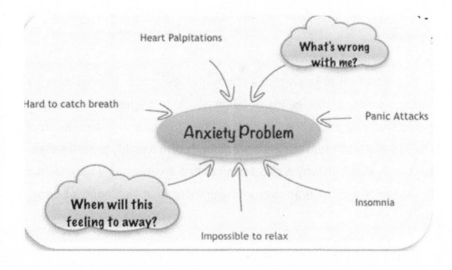

As you can see the 'Anxiety Problem' takes centre-stage in the diagram and links all sorts of anxiety symptoms together. You'll find that a large array of symptoms can surround the core issue of the anxiety problem - particularly those symptoms that feel somewhat 'new' to the person who is experiencing it.

I suggest that at some point, when you feel that you can, you should write down everything that worries you and place all of these worries into an anxiety map like the ones featured here. I honestly can't emphasise enough how such a simple task ends up becoming an enlightening and powerful form of relief. Why not trial pointing your physical and psychological ailments to anxiety? Hopefully you'd have discovered a strong link here.

I, like many others, fell into the trap of assuming the worse about my predicament. *'Something must be wrong with me,'* I often thought, usually spending the majority of my day analysing why I felt the way I did and panicking when the feelings didn't go away. All that I was experiencing was **anxiety** - an unbelievably non-complex condition (despite its many horrible symptoms) that is harmless and easily overcome.

It's important to know that a common feeling that accompanies an anxiety disorder is the feeling of being 'stuck' or trapped in a constant loop of worrying thoughts and panic. When this happens we may start to become anxious for reasons beyond our normal ability to rationalise. We start to dwell on why we feel panicky and are inevitably sucked into the dark world of high anxiety and the increasing likelihood of panic attacks.

Ultimately, we can start to become anxious *because* we are feeling anxious. We can begin to question the very reason why we feel the way we do, and if you're like the 'old' me you probably spend every day doing just this. Every day!

It doesn't take a genius to work out that anxious thoughts and questioning the way you feel can easily become an unwanted, obsessive hobby. You're probably doing it now, or it's queued in your thought pattern somewhere.

This obsessive behaviour can easily spill over and dictate our actions too. Perhaps you've spent days on end perilously researching your symptoms on search engines, only to find that you've been frightened by what you've discovered despite the obvious improbability of it. When we are anxious, we become vulnerable and are easily drawn to the worst-case scenario in a given situation. Search engines often have the habit of churning out fatalistic diagnoses and stories of isolated misfortune. Unfortunately, when we are vulnerable, we are drawn to this information which provides the negativity that feeds our obsessions.

I know it's extremely hard to put scary and repetitive thoughts aside but for now at least, just let it go. Nothing bad will happen to you. 'Bad' is a subjective term, but I deem 'bad' in relation to the topic of anxiety to be the feeling that you're about to die, or something awful is about to happen. Always remember that feeling anxious cannot do this to you.

A common problem with anxiety is that it feels like it's tailored to the individual. The longer the strange feelings and symptoms continue, the more likely we are to assume something is wrong upstairs. By 'upstairs' I mean our constantly ticking, never-resting brains. One day we're feeling fine, then the next day we feel completely different and the world around us also feels and appears different. We fall prey to our feelings and emotions and our reality becomes a superficial projection of what's actually going on.

I, like many others I have helped and who have likewise helped me, found it such a relief to be able to identify and relate to the symptoms which can occur with anxiety. Some of these symptoms present as very strange ones and may have you questioning both why and if they even relate to anxiety at all. The simple answer is that when we are in an anxious state, our body operates on a different level, and over time this different 'mode' of operation takes its toll on the body and mind.

This is all to do with adrenaline and other body chemicals which will be explained in more depth later on. Rest assured, these symptoms are common, and to further ease your worries I have set out a chapter later in this book dedicated to explaining each symptom to you.

The Anxiety Umbrella

The first step any anxiety sufferer should take is to simplify their chaotic world of worries. It unfortunately took me three years to work this out - something that will take you the duration of an afternoon - but rest assured it helped massively in taming my constant worry. It's the first step that should be taken when beginning to assume control of anxiety.

When anxiety is high and blinding confusion has set in, you'll know that it can be extremely difficult to prioritise, organise and focus on your 'problems' in any logical order or with any rational sense. We have so many different worries, which mount up on top of our underlying worry of 'not feeling right', that we simply just don't know where to start. Have you tried waiting for the feelings to go away? You'll know it simply does not work like that.

Take a look at these examples of types of worries below:

Daily Life Worries	Social Worries	Worries from Perspective
• Work / Job • Bills • Finance • Education • Domestic Jobs • Appointments • Security • Deadlines • Examinations • Unenjoyable tasks. • Chores	• Relationships • Friendships • Family • Parenthood • Social Circles • Confidence • Loss of Sense of Humour • Expectations • Judgement	• Religious perspective • Philosophical outlook • Life purpose/meaning • Self Worth • Over analysing situations • Misanthropy • *'The outside world is a scary place'* • *'Nobody understands what I'm going through'*

Hypochondria (Health Worries)

- *'Am I going insane?'*
- Self analysing
- Body checking for problems.
- Fear of having a panic attack
- Convinced of having a heart problem, cancer, schizophrenia etc

Now let's scatter a few examples around in a similar fashion to the anxiety maps. I once again suggest that you take this opportunity to use your own experiences whilst utilising these examples as guides.

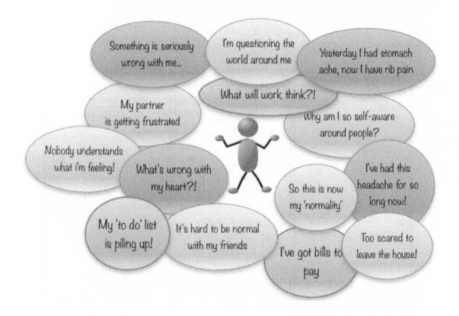

Can you see how hard it must be to prioritise one single worry from out of the many? Where do we even start?

Of course, it's normal to have every day worries such as work and social issues, however these worries can soon multiply and increase in intensity when anxiety is present. Anxiety can soon act as a barrier to resolving every day issues, which results in worries building up very quickly. Worries and stress become harder to resolve causing an accumulation effect similar to that of the common snowball analogy.

The key here, which forms one of the core foundations of this book, is to group everything as one problem - the problem being the simplified term 'anxiety'. Take everything that you've ever assumed and worried about with regards to how you feel and throw it under a metaphorical umbrella. Label it 'anxiety' and voilà – your problems are simplified to one manageable problem.

'*What do I do with this umbrella?*' you may ask. Well, I've written this book to tell you. If I'd have known all that time ago that all I was experiencing were symptoms of anxiety I'd have saved myself a hell of a lot of time and energy. Five years' worth of time to be precise.

Let us take a look at this poorly-drawn anxiety umbrella for some clarity (drawing is not my forte by the way):

The Anxiety Umbrella

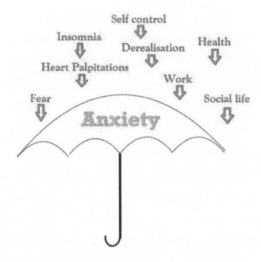

As you can see, the umbrella symbolises anxiety as a whole and the 'rain drops' symbolise some of the components or symptoms that form an anxiety condition. Instead of trying to deal with every issue or symptom separately, I challenge you to try and allow all of your worries to be associated with anxiety. This not only simplifies the problem, it allows room for reflection and for a 'point of blame' if life simply becomes too much.

I'm handing out labels and pills. Who wants some?

In the introduction I referred to the term 'anxiety' from a more generalised perspective when, in fact, it acts as more of a generic name for a plethora of conditions which fall under several different subcategories. Here is a list of conditions which will most likely seem familiar to you either right now or in the future:

- Generalised Anxiety Disorder (GAD)
- Panic Disorder
- Health Anxiety Disorder
- Obsessive Compulsive Disorder
- Anxiety and Depressive Disorder
- Agoraphobia
- Social Anxiety
- Retroactive Jealousy

Of course, there are other strands of anxiety that fall under different categories, but the list above consists of the names that tend to float around the most. Furthermore, I can openly admit that each of the labels listed could, at one time, be associated as a condition that I have personally experienced and been through.

We sometimes put labels on ourselves to provide some false sense of understanding about what we're confused about. It acts as a comfort blanket and simplifies complex issues that we're unsure of or uneducated in. I'm not boldly stating that you have been misdiagnosed, and that I am contradicting the views of a trained medical professional, but what's remarkable about what I have found in my research is the importance sufferers place on possessing a medical label to make sense of what only *appears* to be a complex problem.

A large proportion of the anxiety sufferers I have worked with use these labels to make sense of something they fear, therefore taking the 'edge' off an issue that they find incredibly scary. Look at these for example:

- "I can't go outside because I suffer from *Agoraphobia*"
- "I have a *Panic Disorder* so I can't attend the event"
- "When this *Depression* leaves I can return to my normal life"
- "I wish I could do all these things but I have an *Anxiety Disorder*"
- "Don't blame me it's my *O.C.D*"

So... if you can relate to anything this book has mentioned so far then I throw down the gauntlet to you - I dare you to lose any labels you've attributed to yourself and simply blame everything on anxiety. The advantage of openly acknowledging you have an anxiety 'condition' is that a condition can be changed. It is merely temporary.

You could argue that acknowledging you have an anxiety condition is much like giving yourself a new label. However, I'm asking you to acknowledge anxiety as a changeable condition – one that can be immediately challenged and laid to rest.

The first thing I had to do to tackle my anxiety was to lose the labels I held above my head and structured my life around. I *knew* I was depressed, I *knew* I was scared to leave the house and I *knew* things were a lot different from before.

What I realised was that it wasn't the medical condition crippling me, but the constant and overwhelming *fear* that overcame me on a daily basis. After much deep thought I decided that if a medical condition was to dictate my life it could do so, but I was in no way going to let my life be dictated by a negative emotion. Fear was not going to dictate my life. Fear is an emotion, not a medical condition.

An anxiety problem can be fixed with understanding and good practice; before long you'll be living a life free from the clutches of gripping fear and worry. I sit here today laughing at the years I spent trapped in this loop of high anxiety and panic, but at the same time I know that I could have saved years of my life if I had been educated earlier.

This is where I feel a lot of people's problems lie, in terms of their anxiety getting out of hand. Focusing on the health profession's role within the world of anxiety it is in my and many others' opinion that (while acknowledging the excellent work done by many in the profession and within mental health) certain sectors of the health profession approach anxiety with too much haste and misunderstanding. Many people feel that the common referral processes, combined with an overloaded demand for access to services, can often lead to misdiagnosis, mistreatment and a lack of time assessing the individual and their needs.

Perhaps like me you've sampled the many medicinal approaches to treating anxiety such as anti-depressants, pseudo drugs, herbal remedies and 'miracle cures'. Once again, I'm not in a position to state the positive benefits of such medicines, but what I can share with you is that I, together with many others I have helped, found that these drugs did not help at all in terms of easing the symptoms of anxiety and the underlying fear that accompanies it.

Drugs such as anti-depressants are undoubtedly designed to change how we feel. When we are anxious we are vulnerable to states of hypersensitivity - meaning that we're alert to any change in ourselves and our environment. This is why it's commonly found that anti-depressants don't allow anxiety victims to get to the core of the problem. We often spend a lot of time scanning ourselves to see if we're 'okay', but with drugs altering our current state of mind they can often end up causing the opposite of the intended outcome. We panic and over-think about everything that seems different within or around us. Ultimately, they can heighten our sense of *losing control*.

I trust my general practitioner, and my CBT nurse, but overall I think the medical profession lacks the knowledge about the topic of anxiety as a whole and are too quick to throw pills at it alongside grouping it with depression. Anxiety is not depression. Anxiety can only lead to depression over time, or when someone has assumed that their future lies in only ever feeling a certain way.

This is the reason behind writing this book. The answer to conquering your anxiety is pretty simple but has overwhelming results. All I ask of you is to ask yourself *'Do I have all of these separate problems?'* or, is it simply a question of *'Do I have an anxiety problem.*

1.2 Why am I panicking and where did this come from?

Constant overwhelming anxiety, quite unsurprisingly, is caused by the sufferer getting into the habit of too much worry. Over time excessive and continual worry creates a chemical imbalance within our bodies causing constant, unmeasured amounts of adrenaline and other chemicals to be released into our systems. These chemicals, in any measure, can and *will* cause noticeable changes in us both physically and mentally - particularly when adrenaline is released in large amounts on a frequent basis.

It's important to explain that quite often our biggest worry during these times is the constant awareness of feeling different from our usual selves and in a lot of cases feeling a detachment from our surroundings. This is called entering states of *depersonalization* and *derealisation*. These symptoms can be extremely discomforting and can often leave us feeling frightened. We can find ourselves rapidly foraging for an answer to the newly-found problem - striving for order and an explanation for a feeling that we currently feel clueless about.

Like I mentioned before, the main culprit for these feelings is the wonderful chemical **adrenaline** - with the aid of some other bodily chemicals that get released, such as cortisol. These chemicals are primarily responsible for leading us into episodes of extreme panic, hypersensitivity, lucid derealization, and for triggering concern about other physical symptoms. Adrenaline isn't a chemical to be feared however, it just needs to be understood.

Further to adrenaline affecting our bodies, when anxiety and panic strike frequently and continuously over time, they begin to over-stimulate the nervous system. An over-stimulated nervous system sets us on high alert mode and it's more than common to feel hyperaware, hypersensitive and overly conscious of 'dangers' in our surroundings and even within our bodies. It's easy to become overly *aware* of our anxiety, our panic and how different we currently feel from our usual selves.

I realise that up to now there's a lot to take in, so let's break it down. Go to the next page for a simplified break down.

Breaking it down:

- Poor thought patterns and a bad behavioral routine cause the body to release excessive amounts of adrenaline.

- Adrenaline causes various changes within our bodies and eventually causes a chemical imbalance.

- Over time a constant flow of adrenaline causes us to become hypersensitive and hyperaware of ourselves and our surroundings (Fight or Flight response).

- Adrenaline and hypersensitivity can cause us to experience episodes of depersonalisation and derealisation.

- Over time our nervous systems become over-stimulated making us further prone to anxiety and panic. We begin to panic about why we feel the way we do.

- We begin to panic about the other symptoms anxiety can cause (refer to symptoms list).

- We're stuck in a loop of worrying and panicking about our well-being and attaching our own reasoning to why we feel the way we do.

It may sound unmeasured, but all you need to know is that you have an **anxiety problem**. Or to put it in other words, you're failing to understand and accept what adrenaline is doing to your body. I suspect that almost all of your problems revolve around how you and your body react to dumps of adrenaline and how you re-enact negative thought and behaviour habits.

Of course, everyone experiences doses of adrenaline on a frequent basis. It is a normal bodily chemical that helps us function as human beings by triggering our 'fight or flight' response. However, when it becomes excessive - particularly when caused by stress, negative thoughts and behaviours - it can easily turn into a daily anxiety or panic problem. Instead of our days being 'normal' they can turn into prolonged battles against our own minds and bodies which is nothing short of exhausting.

It is of absolute importance to understand and accept that an anxiety problem and frequent panic attacks don't just occur overnight; they are the result of something that has built up over time. This could have been started by worrying about personal and subjective issues, or triggered by a life event causing a traumatic effect on the body.

When these worries aren't dealt with or solved, they then unknowingly accumulate on top of one another causing the sufferer to reach their peak in terms of being in an anxious state. The sufferer (you) is stuck in a constant fluctuation between high anxiety and panic.

These worries then often evolve into *new* worries that revolve around well-being and the concept of suffering from a mental health condition, i.e. 'going insane'. Free-flowing adrenaline is being released in copious amounts - causing all sorts of changes both physically and mentally - and we're left in a bit of a mess. The next section goes into this in more detail.

But wait a second! A pretty grounded person would be intelligent enough to work out these feelings and emotions themselves, so why not do just that?

No, this would be a colossal error.

It's a common trap for many people when acknowledging something is wrong to then attempt to use seemingly harmless logic to try to 'solve' the anxiety problem. Another common trap is to simply wait for the feelings to go away.

'Working it out' is just another worry added onto the giant *smorgasbord* of worries that we previously had. Panic then sets in because we have waited more than enough time for these feelings to disappear, but alas they linger and appear to become stronger than ever!

Then, to make things even more complicated, the physical symptoms that come hand-in-hand with worry start to appear. The headaches, stomach cramps, reality distortion, racing heart beats, shortness of breath, dizziness and sweating to name a mere few. What an even greater mess!

Fight-or-Flight

A physiological reaction in response to stress, characterized by an increase in heart rate and blood pressure, elevation of glucose levels in the blood, and redistribution of blood from the digestive tract to the muscles. These changes are caused by activation of the sympathetic nervous system by epinephrine (adrenaline), which prepares the body to challenge or flee from a perceived threat.

-The American Heritage® Science Dictionary

To put it simply, our anxiety is caused by a simple imbalance in the body caused by continuous stress or trauma. Adrenaline and other chemicals are released in disproportionate amounts causing us to feel strange and hypersensitive to aches, pains, other bodily changes and what's happening in our environment. Our nervous systems become over-stimulated, which further puts us on high alert and makes us sensitive to changes in ourselves and our environment. However, as many of us are unaware of this, we are stuck worrying and questioning the way we feel and why we feel so scared. We become victims to our own hypersensitivity.

The Loop of Peaking Anxiety

It is extremely important to understand that you don't just wake up with full blown anxiety. It is a condition that reveals its true colours over time and is often only consciously identifiable at its **peak**. This means that the working cogs of your anxiety condition were put into motion at some point in the past and it is only now that you are aware that something is wrong because your anxiety is *peaking*.

This would explain why anxiety and panic attacks crop up from seemingly nowhere (my first panic attack struck when I was making a cup of tea at work). The peak of anxiety is often represented by sudden waves of anxiety, panic and an onslaught of the symptoms mentioned at the start of this book. These symptoms can be ever present, they can also 'come and go', or they can be completely new to the sufferer as a result of a stressful week.

The overall result is a *loop* of anxious thoughts and relentless worry - something which I have labeled **The Loop of Peaking Anxiety**. I will use this diagram to provide more clarity.

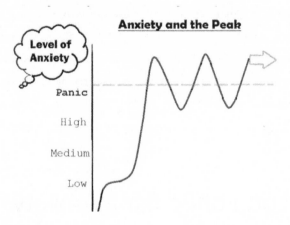

Anything below the ***Medium*** level you would class as 'normal' anxiety - the worries that warrant an anxious response to issues found on a day-to-day basis. Note that even a high level of anxiety is normal, but when our anxiety exceeds this we are at risk of being struck with **panic**.

Unfortunately, it is common for many anxiety victims to be stuck fluctuating between high anxiety and panic, with the result being a traumatic 'loop' effect. Suddenly the normal day-to-day worries are not at the forefront of priorities anymore, with but replaced by worries about our well-being and this newly formed anxious state.

Consider the following analogy:

Imagine your anxiety being channeled through an electrical plug. The electrical plug has a fuse which represents your body's **coping mechanisms**. The more stress and worrying thoughts that you pile on yourself, then the stronger the power the plug's fuse has to deal with.

The stress and worry slowly builds up until your body simply can't take anymore. The fuse blows, the circuit shuts down and you're left in a confused mess trying to work out what exactly just happened. You can't operate like you used to anymore because there is nothing to control all of this surging 'power'.

The body's coping mechanisms - which consist of positive rationalisation, your body's ability to maintain a chemical balance and the familiar feeling of accepting what you're used to – have completely gone, thus unveiling a bizarre world of terror and confusion. You are left to work out an answer to an unsolvable puzzle. You start to question why you feel the way you do, *why* it happened, finding your own irrational solutions etc. You can become stuck within the infamous loop! Fear not, as this is easily fixed with the power of understanding.

To the unaware sufferer it can be very difficult to 'return' or settle down to normality again. It's not uncommon that people have lived with anxiety for years, stuck in the same looping habit of questioning why they feel the way they do, or just waiting for the feelings and thoughts to disappear.

Many victims, including myself at one time, make it a depressing routine to constantly self-analyse – first checking how we feel, then scanning our bodies for signs that there is something wrong. We do this because we're stuck in the *loop of peaking anxiety*.

We often resign ourselves to thinking we have an incurable, psychological condition because frankly we often conclude that nothing seems to be working. What we don't fully realise is that we're thinking out of *fear* and consciously looking for reasons to provide fabrication and meaning for this fear. One of the worst mistakes I made was to wake up and immediately think *"Do I feel better today?!"* Funnily enough I didn't.

Being stuck in a loop at the peak of your anxiety is debilitating, depressing and awfully scary. However, use the knowledge of why you feel this way to provide a small, comforting degree of inner content. You are not going insane and in fact <u>what you're experiencing is alarmingly common</u>. What's also reassuring is that what your body is doing is only natural, so no matter how long you've had this condition I can repeat my earlier assurances that nothing 'bad' will happen to you as a result of it. You could be anxious for the next one hundred years and your death would not be directly anxiety related.

No matter how many times you lose your breath, feel your heart pounding, lose your balance, feel lightheaded or focus on an abnormality - remember that the anxiety will not kill you. Anxiety is harmless and merely tricks you into thinking the world is crumbling around you and that you're dying a depressing, isolated death.

Part 1.3 explains what's exactly happening to you and your body during episodes of high anxiety and panic. With the power of understanding you will realise that what is happening does not warrant the fear that accompanies it.

Why does an anxiety problem start?

There are two simple reasons why anxiety starts and later becomes horribly excessive:

The first cause is a basic one and that's human habit. When we get into a habit of worrying and constantly troubling ourselves with undesirable thoughts, this eventually takes its toll on the body. Have you ever been labeled a 'worrier'? Or know somebody in your life who you would deem to be a worrier?

Cognitive Behavioural Therapy tells us that obsessive worrying about certain thoughts is just the inability to detach from or let go of a thought. If you cannot let go or lessen the importance of a thought, then the worry that accompanies it simply sticks around striving for attention and piling up with other worries.

We get into a habit of worrying until the body becomes disturbed, causing all of this anxiety and its army of symptoms to appear. It took a very long time for me to acknowledge and admit to myself that I was a worrier. It required me to study my thought patterns for a long time.

The second cause is trauma. Trauma starts the anxiety problem in a similar fashion to the first cause, except that it skips the build-up and gives your body a raging fireball to deal with. Referring back to the preceding analogy, trauma basically tries pushing the equivalent of the national grid through the 'plug socket' causing an immediate blow-out.

Trauma is usually started by an unexpected incident in life where the body is put into shock. I.e., the death of a loved one, personal injury or illness, exposure to a fear, loss of job, divorce, adultery, and so on. Your coping mechanisms are wiped out and become non-existent. You perceive life differently compared with before the trauma, and unsurprisingly your body has a major chemical imbalance. You feel different and of course you now want to know why.

It's an extremely important part of your recovery to acknowledge exactly where the anxiety has come from and why it is happening to you. It takes a lot of bravery to admit to yourself that perhaps you were doing something self-inflicting - particularly if you're a pretty self-assured person who thinks you have a large degree of self-control in your life.

I unfortunately developed my anxiety as a young man with a pretty large ego. What I failed to acknowledge is that my thought patterns were very negative and damaging in terms of affecting my mental health. I developed anxiety as a result of a poor mental routine and then eventually having to deal with a shocking life event. I will explain more about my story later on in this book.

1.3 Anxiety is Adrenaline and a Sensitive Nervous System

I think the most influential factor in my recovery was forming an understanding of what was actually happening during the episodes of high anxiety and panic. Of course, I was aware of the more obvious related symptoms such as the racing thoughts, a fast heart rate, difficulty maintaining steady breathing, light headedness and the odd aches and pains. But the real panic came from wondering where these symptoms actually came from and *why* they were happening to me.

Unfortunately, I made the ultimate mistake of falling into one of anxiety's most formidable traps. I began to *fear* anxiety. I began to fear feeling panicky and feeling different - something which firmly fixes you within the clutches of anxiety.

In section 1.2, I explained about how anxiety builds up, and how our bodies react to these anxious and frightening thoughts by releasing chemicals such as adrenaline and cortisol.

Adrenaline is a funny little chemical. It is great in times of danger and acts as a great defence mechanism for the body by triggering our 'fight or flight' response. However, when we are stuck in a habit of dwelling on frightening thoughts in a situation where 'fight or flight' isn't needed, then adrenaline seems to become our adversary.

Our brain and adrenal gland start to work together by releasing plenteous amounts of adrenaline at times where we don't *need* it - thus causing our bodies to react to the adrenaline, causing all of these strange symptoms to appear and temporarily alter our perception of reality. It is the *thoughts* that keep triggering the adrenal gland to release these chemicals. It is the negative thoughts - not the will for the feeling to stop - that keep the adrenaline pumping.

Think about it! Can you recall how you felt the last time you dealt with a large dose of adrenaline? Try and recall how much you were stuck in your own head the minutes before a job interview, a risky operation or even something leisurely like a first date. Adrenaline is pumping through your system and all you seem to focus on is the situation that is imminent and directly in front of you. It's exactly the same when we are stuck with an anxiety problem.

Adrenaline and other bodily chemicals swim around our veins - affecting everything that we're used to during a 'normal' day - and we're left worrying and questioning why we feel so different and *why* we are constantly worrying. There appears to be no plausible danger in front of us, yet our body prepares us for one by constantly triggering the 'fight or flight' response. This inevitably led me, for one, to become stuck in the 'Loop of Peaking Anxiety'. Never underestimate the power of thoughts and how they affect the body over time.

Constantly worrying about why I felt the way I did just led to my body constantly releasing adrenaline into the bloodstream. Over time the worry inevitably led to the intense presence of stress both mentally and physically. This caused yet more worry because I then started to focus on the physical changes my body was going through.

Adrenaline causes all sorts of changes within the body, and over time it's usually responsible for all sorts of weird and wonderful things that can occur. It is extremely important to know that, in relation to anxiety, continuous adrenaline can be found to be primarily responsible for:

- Increase in heart rate / palpitations / pounding chest ("Fight or Flight")

- Sudden and continuous sense of derealisation/ detachment from surroundings
- Racing, looping thoughts ("Fight or Flight")
- Difficulty maintaining steady breathing/ shortness of breath ("Fight or Flight")
- Dizziness / light headedness / vision distortion
- Excessive sweating / hot flushes
- Muscle tension ("Fight or Flight")
- Hypersensitivity
- Panic attacks

I recall dwelling on constant headaches, abdominal pains, lack of sleep and why my surroundings felt detached from me. Furthermore, I used to focus obsessively on an array of symptoms found in the **symptom list** at the start of the book. Everything felt different from what it used to be like and I needed to know why. The difficulty was that I didn't accept that these feelings would only be temporary if I allowed the adrenaline and cortisol to run its course and let my body restore a chemical balance.

The solution that we strive for is so simple, but we can all fall victim to our racing thoughts and pay too much attention to them. If we just allow adrenaline to run its course, then the feeling of normality will eventually return. 'Normality' returns faster and faster the more we get used to paying our negative thoughts and feelings zero attention.

Panic Attacks

When anxiety is at its highest - where worrying thoughts, stress, tiredness and a damaging routine have taken their toll - we experience something called a panic attack. A panic attack can also occur when we are exposed to shock, sudden trauma or anything that scares us.

A lot of people use the term as a means of exaggeration when in conversation. For example, *'Wow you scared me! You almost gave me a panic attack!'* would undoubtedly be something that you've heard in your lifetime. An actual panic attack however feels nothing short of terrifying to the person who is experiencing it.

A panic attack is when an intense feeling of fear, dread, loss of control and entrapment overwhelms a person. There is usually no identifiable trigger and they seem to strike from *seemingly* nowhere (you have learned that this is untrue). Accompanying these feelings are thoughts of imminent disaster, impending doom and even the fear of sudden death. The number of anxiety victims I have spoken to who have ended up in the emergency room with no explainable symptoms borders on the absurd!

A panic attack leads you down roads of irrational thinking, where even the most intelligent of people are forced to feel and believe in the most unlikely of outcomes. I used to whirl up in a panic over a chest flutter, headache, differences in breathing, stomach cramps, detachment from surroundings . Along with these feelings are other physical symptoms that occur when panic has struck. A panic attack causes our muscles to tense up, our peripheral vision to shut down (tunnel vision) and alters the way we breath - tricking us into thinking we're not getting enough oxygen. It also causes light headedness, dizziness and sometimes nausea. Below are the main symptoms and feelings that occur during a panic attack, some of which have already appeared in other earlier lists.

Panic Attacks

- Sudden and intense fright.
- A sense of derealisation / detachment from surroundings.
- Chest pains.
- Pounding or thumping chest.
- Fast heart rate.
- Difficulty maintaining a steady pace of breathing.
- An overwhelming urge to 'escape' or run away.
- Irrational thinking. I.e. *Am I going to die? Is this a heart attack? I must have a serious condition like cancer.*
- Chest fluttering / heart palpitations.
- Racing thoughts and confusion.
- The urge to do anything but be stationary i.e. pace the room or squeeze an object.
- Tunnel Vision.

A panic attack can occur when the body releases a large amount of unexpected adrenaline into the bloodstream. I mentioned before that adrenaline can cause all sorts of changes both physically and mentally, so if we're unprepared or 'caught off-guard' by a newly-released dump of adrenaline, then it could be expected that we panic about this sudden change.

The panic comes from the **confusion** about what is happening and this works in tandem with a belief that you can no longer cope. Adrenaline actually causes our minds to race and be filled with all sorts of thoughts and conclusions as to *why* we're panicking and *why* we're feeling strange.

This would explain why so many people are convinced that they're having a heart attack, or that they're going insane, or that they have an incurable condition, and so on. It is the adrenaline that affects our rationality during these periods of panic, thus causing them to turn into prolonged *panic attacks.*

These panic attacks don't last forever because the adrenal gland finally becomes exhausted and cannot release any further adrenaline. The reader should take comfort in the fact that a panic attack cannot last forever because of this and the feeling of normality will return - at least until the adrenal gland has recharged and we may unknowingly fall back into the same repetitive thought habit.

Let's take a look at the *Anxiety and the Peak* diagram from 1.1 and explore how panic attacks tie in with the loop of peaking anxiety:

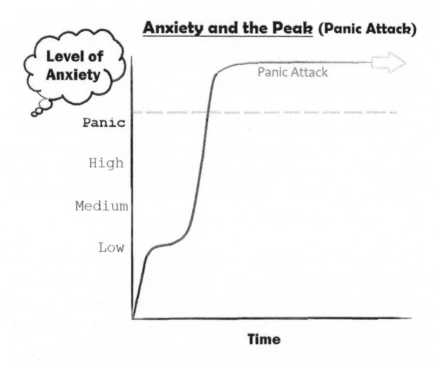

Anxiety and the Peak (Panic Attack)

Instead of our anxiety and panic 'looping', a panic attack occurs when we're struck with a feeling of constant fear. To the person who experiences it the feeling can often feel like the fear is escalating or 'getting worse'. This is purely psychosomatic because a panic attack occurs at the peak of an adrenal outpour. In other words, and on a comforting note, once you're having a panic attack it can't get any 'worse' than when it initially struck.

I, like many others, suffered my first panic attack in a situation where it appeared to creep up from 'nowhere'. I was on my break at work, pouring myself a cup of tea, when I was suddenly struck and overwhelmed by a feeling of detachment from my surroundings. My breathing started to alter and I immediately felt worried as this feeling seemed so different to me. I inevitably started to panic; then I started to panic because I didn't know why I was panicking. I wanted normality to come straight back to me because I didn't feel in control of a situation that I was usually in complete control of.

Simply put, a panic attack is just a reaction to an unwanted dose of adrenaline. Stress, anxiety, fatigue, poor diet and lack of sleep lead to an imbalance within the body and our nervous systems become over-stimulated. This causes adrenaline to be released after the slightest, almost unnoticeable, trigger.

Use this knowledge and I assure you the next panic attack will not be half as bad. Since I learned this, the panic attacks became less and less intense and the duration decreased over a relatively short amount of time. I will provide further information and advice on dealing with panic attacks in the next part of this book.

Rationality and Worst-Case Scenarios

One of the most profound stumbling blocks that occur when trying to tackle anxiety is that of falling prey to our emotions and states of irrationality. When high states of panic and anxiety arise, a common thing we do as human beings is to try to work out what exactly is happening in order to make sense of a situation that can appear very confusing.

It is extremely important to acknowledge that when anxiety is present, our normal sense of what is rational can be massively distorted. Our thinking can become predominantly irrational due to the adrenaline that's flowing through our veins and implementing change in our bodies. We can become frightened at the possibility of something horrendous happening in any given situation. Trying to think rationally in 'fight or flight' mode is extremely tricky.

Take these scenarios as examples: you're at home alone at night and you hear a loud bang, the first thing that commonly comes to mind is thinking is there an intruder in the house? Other examples that lead to irrational thinking include the scenario where your child does not come home on time, or the boss calls you in for an unexpected meeting.

We are plagued by the frightening thoughts of our child being abducted, or the boss handing us our notice. When thinking about these situations using a calm sense of rationality, we could come to the more likely conclusions that the nighttime noise was actually just a falling object, and that our child's bus is only running late, and the boss just wants to give us a new task relating to work.

These situations are usually resolved in due time and we commonly enter a quick state of relief due to these frightening possibilities not becoming a reality. However, this is where anxiety can cripple us. Anxiety can seemingly force us into believing irrational scenarios (such as those mentioned above) even when we aren't faced with such scenarios. We can begin to fabricate our own scenarios with our own devised, variable outcomes for that given situation. Let me explain further.

Say for example we were suffering from a persistent headache, but we *didn't* suffer from an anxiety problem. Our thought spread may look similar to this:

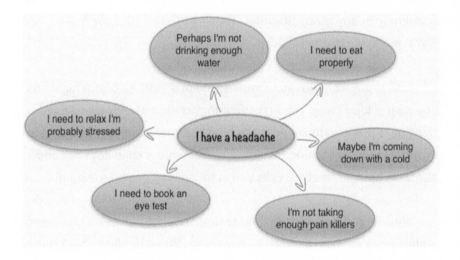

Each of the thought conclusions represents a common form of rationale with at least one of them likely to be the answer or 'solution'. Using a balanced sense of rationale we can almost conclude that the cause of the headache is down to one of the thoughts/possibilities above. Everyone experiences headaches at some point and they are almost always no cause for immediate concern.

Now let us look at how a high state of anxiety can affect a person's use of rationale using the same headache scenario. Below is another thought spread, this time representing how anxiety can cause us to believe in the scariest but unlikeliest of scenarios:

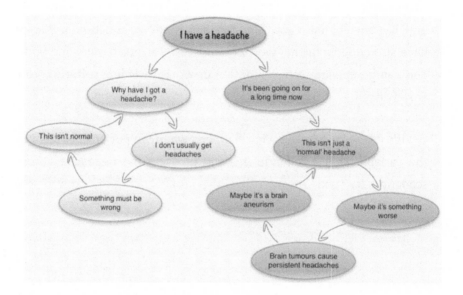

Look at how anxiety can distort and change the thinking process when dealing with an everyday scenario. The first headache scenario shows how a calm sense of rational thinking can help us find a quick conclusion to a situation. However, the one above represents something as simple as a headache quickly developing into an anxious problem. The headache in this situation has now turned into a worry and thus has caused *more* anxiety.

The thinking process in the second diagram actually creates a twofold problem. When we are anxious we look to attach reasoning to the anxiety to help us understand why we feel the way we do. The more extreme the anxiety, then the more extreme the worst-case scenario appears to be.

To continue the example, the headache is assumed to be something that's potentially dangerous and frightening - a worst-case scenario. Not only has anxiety led us to this scary and irrational conclusion, but we have also added a further worry to an already stressed mind and body. This can be applied to any situation or worry including suffering from anxiety itself.

It's interesting to see what happens when we put anxiety itself as the variable in our scenario. Instead of using the headache as our scenario, try and replace it with 'adrenaline' and explore the possibilities.

PART 2

Anxiety Symptoms Explained

THIS SECTION OF THE book provides explanations for the symptoms that are associated with having an ongoing anxiety condition. Here you will find an itemised encyclopedic-style symptoms list, along with explanations as to why and how these symptoms can be caused by anxiety. There will undoubtedly be symptoms that will not relate to you, but I certainly recommend that you to read through them all so that you're well equipped if they ever occur in the future.

The information provided here derives from a combination of personal experience and observational research about the topic of anxiety, but is in no way official medical print or to be prioritised over the opinion of a health professional. Having said this, I am extremely confident in stating that each symptom found here has a direct link to anxiety and the likelihood of the symptoms being caused or aggravated by anxiety is, in my opinion, unquestionable.

The symptoms list at the start of this book separates the symptoms into two lists – the **psychological symptoms** and the **physical symptoms**. In this part of the book I have ordered the symptoms list starting with the most commonly occurring symptoms, then moving towards the more obscure symptoms.

You will find that the explanations for certain symptoms will sound familiar or relate to other listed symptoms. This is due to anxiety and its symptoms all being linked together, which in itself is a positive in terms of simplifying everything and recognising that we have an anxiety problem - much like the *anxiety umbrella*.

2.1 Derealisation / detachment / 'feeling weird'

What? This occurs in almost everyone who experiences excessive anxiety and panic. Derealisation occurs when our reality and surroundings feel and appear distorted and we become highly aware that we feel 'different' from our usual selves. It's common for many sufferers to feel very lucid at times of derealisation and almost entirely detached from their surroundings. Many have described it as feeling like they are uncomfortably floating, or as if they're existing in a room in third person.

You could, for example, be in a certain place that's very familiar to you, but the natural feelings and recognition associated with the place are missing. Feelings of **vertigo**, **light headedness** and **tunnel vision** are also common when identifying an episode of derealisation. It's important to understand that episodes of derealisation can be responsible for a large number of panic attacks and can often act as the trigger, due to it seeming to appear 'out of nowhere' and being immediately misinterpreted.

People often find it extremely **difficult to relax** at times of derealisation and often fall into the trap of trying to over-think a way out of it. Over time, derealisation can outweigh feelings of normality and can actually present itself for longer periods of time than a 'normal', settled state. This gives the victim a false projection of reality, causing all sorts of problems and swaying a person's perception of the world around them. Feelings of derealisation are completely harmless and will pass with time, patience and a change in behaviour habits.

Why? Derealisation occurs as a result of a stressful routine and an accumulation of negative thoughts and behaviours. It can also appear as the result of trauma. It's a sign that the body's nervous system is hypersensitive and that the body is also currently working on a chemical imbalance by releasing all sorts of chemicals into the blood stream.

Feeling lucid and detached from your surroundings is also an indicator that there is an abnormal amount of adrenaline floating around your system. High amounts of adrenaline cause us to become hypersensitive and it temporarily alters our nervous system - putting us on high alert for signs of a 'problem' or danger, causing us to intricately analyse ourselves and our surroundings.

During episodes of high or abnormally flowing adrenaline, our bodies change in response to the chemical. **Our peripheral vision shuts down**, our **breathing alters** and our ability to **focus becomes difficult**. Feeling detached from our surroundings - particularly when we don't know *why* we feel detached - can be extremely frightening for those who find it hard to deal with a lack of control. However, the feelings inevitably subside as the adrenal gland will either stop releasing as much adrenaline or will eventually exhaust itself.

2.2 Unexplainable fear / fear of going 'insane'

What? Fear is an emotion that becomes embedded within us as we grow up and is also part of our make up as human beings. However, when worry and fear become irrational to the point where they are debilitating to our lives, then they become obvious symptoms related to an anxiety problem. An anxiety condition usually presents itself with episodes of mild to extreme bouts of unexplainable fear. This is due to the body dealing with doses of adrenaline and cortisol which are usually released at times we're not expecting.

Unfortunately, we sometimes try to make sense of this fear by attaching our own fabricated reasons and thoughts to it. Mild fears such as going to the shops, or suffering from a persistent headache, become exaggerated fears which can be moulded to explain why we are feeling so anxious. Going to the shops suddenly becomes too dangerous, and a headache is a clear sign of a brain tumour. Furthermore, this unexplainable fear has been the reason why so many people have taken unnecessary trips to the emergency department, or rung for the emergency services because they are convinced they're having a heart attack or that they're going insane. We try to make sense of the fear by attaching a **worst-case scenario** to explain it. This all ties in with 3.3 in Part 1 - *Rationality and Worst Case Scenarios.*

This fear causes us to take up all sorts of irregular behaviours. This includes **pacing** around a room, finding it **difficult to relax, scanning our body and environment** for 'problems' and **trying to work out *why*** we feel the way we do. The fear can also channel into a person's **fear of panic attacks**.

The fear has always been present, since the evolution of the anxiety problem itself, but because the prospect of having a panic attack is so frightening we can become stuck in the loop of peaking anxiety - *worrying* about having another panic attack. This is another example of attaching reasons to the fear as a means of making sense of it.

Why? As explained above, the intense presence of fear is due to an imbalance within the body and the presence of fear-inducing chemicals such as adrenaline. The imbalance occurs as a result of a poor thought routine, which confuses the brain into thinking - when and where is the best time to become ready to activate the 'fight or flight' response? This would explain why fear can suddenly overwhelm us from nowhere, or that we become unusually fearful of a circumstance that wouldn't usually warrant such a response.

Fear is one of the main barriers that can hinder a positive change when tackling anxiety. Although I, and many other anxiety victims, hated feeling anxious on a daily basis I unfortunately felt a degree of comfort knowing that anxiety was the only constant in my life. I felt that if I tried to change, or do things differently, then I would make my 'condition' worse. Take note that this is completely irrational and borders on the absurd. Fear prevents you from doing things that you have irrationally learned are dangerous. Changing who you are - for the better and for a more positive life - is *not* a dangerous task.

2.3 Hyperventilating / 'I'm not getting enough oxygen'

What? The feeling where breathing becomes an added effort and all of our attention is suddenly focused on our breathing. This can be misconceived as feeling like we're not getting enough oxygen, or it can create a panic reaction because we question why we're breathing so abnormally. Irregular breathing usually occurs when we feel panicky and anxious, but can also happen when we're feeling physically encumbered by things such as stomach bloating or tiredness.

Why? Almost every anxiety sufferer has been concerned about breathing at some point when living with the condition. When we are anxious our heart rate usually increases, so to compensate for this we breathe in more oxygen. Throughout the day we begin to shallow breathe because the anxiety has caused us to take in more oxygen than is required. However, many mis-take this natural shallow breathing as the feeling that we're not getting enough oxygen, so we then begin to breathe in more – and we begin to hyperventilate. The body can't produce the carbon dioxide it needs to get rid of in time, so we find ourselves hyperventilating for quite a while.

During a **panic attack** it's very common for someone to hyperventilate and it can often prolong the panic attack. That's why so much importance is placed on breathing when dealing with anxiety and panic. Shallow breathing can also be responsible for other anxiety symptoms, such as: **heart palpitations, chest pains, feeling lightheaded and dizzy**. It can also alter the way we think and **cause difficulty when trying to focus**.

The short-term benefits of controlling our breathing are helpful and that's why they're promoted so widely, but I personally feel that too much importance is placed on trying to 'control' the breathing because it can apply heavy pressure on the anxiety sufferer. When we are anxious it is common to be very **self-aware/hypersensitive** to any changes or abnormalities that occur in our bodies. I feel that focusing on abnormal breathing often creates a negative effect, as it can lead to panic and hyperventilation. Although it causes other symptoms, shallow breathing isn't particularly dangerous and you'll actually find that it 'disappears' when you deal with the core of the problem. It's an anxiety problem, not a breathing problem.

2.4 Heart palpitations / flutters / 'skipping a beat'

What? I have found that almost every anxiety sufferer - including myself at the time of writing this book - experiences sensations and differences in the rhythm of the heart at times. Heart palpitations are a sudden fast beating of the heart that seems to occur either unexpectedly, after some form of physical exertion, or triggered by a negative thought. They can happen as frequently as every day, every week or just once in a while. Heart palpitations can also present themselves as a **fluttering sensation** in the chest and sternum area, and also the feeling that your heart has **'skipped a beat'**.

Heart palpitations can happen to anyone and usually pass unnoticed in the majority of people. However, they can intensify and increase in frequency when they're considered a problem by the average anxiety sufferer. The process of worrying about heart palpitations creates a *catch 22* situation; the more we worry about the palpitations specifically, then the more frequently they seem to occur.

The link between worrying specifically about the palpitations and the frequency of them isn't mutually inclusive, but when we do persistently worry about them we are easily lead into states of **hyperawareness** because we fear them occurring again. We succeed in noticing and living through every noticeable change in the rhythm of the heart - even those that are natural and occur every day in almost everybody. This is called being left in a **state of apprehension**, which causes our bodies to become **tense** and we're ultimately left in an irrational **state of hypersensitivity** waiting for the next **palpation/flutter/skipping a beat** to happen again.

Why? There are various reasons why differences in the rhythm of the heart can occur. Heart palpitations, chest flutters and temporary irregular beating are found to be very common with anxiety and are almost certainly not a sign of a serious heart condition (please see a health professional if you have doubts). There are many causes that trigger a heart palpitation, not all of which can be identified prior to a palpitation occurring. Some of the most common causes are down to:

- A surge of released adrenaline
- An electrolyte imbalance
- Hormonal changes
- Too much oxygen
- Physical exertion
- Change and fluctuations in blood pressure
- Anxious thoughts
- Diet factors e.g. caffeine, sugar intake, nicotine
- Dehydration
- Periods / Menstrual cycle
- Medication

I used to suffer from palpitations on a daily basis and over time they began to calm down as I focused on my initial reaction to them. I taught myself that they weren't going to cause me any harm and that although they were scary, it was ultimately down to factors associated with my anxiety that were causing them. To help further my aim I changed my diet, quit smoking, cut out caffeine and drank more water.

Notably, I found through my research and the collaborative views of others that all of the causes listed above are linked in some way to being anxious - either physically or psychologically. First, stress and anxiety often cause us to make drastic changes to our diet. It's common for an anxiety sufferer to **search for 'escapes'**, or temporary relief, through things such as alcohol, fatty comfort foods and smoking. We are perhaps led to eating drastically more or considerably less, and our water intake maybe differs from our usual consumption. Diet factors, stress, medication and dehydration can all make differences to our blood pressure, which in turn causes further noticeable changes in our bodies - including changes to the rhythm of the heart.

Our electrolyte levels are altered by the physical symptoms of anxiety, physical exertion, lack of nutrients from our diet and dehydration. We lose electrolytes through our sweat - either through exercise or sweating when we're anxious or panicking. An electrolyte imbalance is often a cause of palpitations occurring, which can be fixed with an improved diet and adequate hydration. Then of course the most common causes of heart palpitations in anxiety sufferers are the **surges of adrenaline** that seem to occur at any time of day. An adrenal and hormonal imbalance directly affects the heart rate but is actually harmless, and becomes less frequent when the sufferer comes to terms with the condition.

Chest flutters aren't always linked to the heart and are often misinterpreted as the heart 'fluttering' or beating quickly. **Acid reflux, trapped wind, I.B.S** and **indigestion** often release gastrointestinal gases and create excess stomach acid, which can apply pressure to the chest and sternum area causing a 'fluttering' affect. This will be explained more later under *Irritable Bowel Syndrome.* Flutters can also be mistaken for **spasms in the chest muscles**, which are another very common symptom of anxiety.

2.5 Chest pains

What? Anxiety can often cause the victim to feel various pains that can occur in and across the chest area. It's important to note that these pains can alter in the way they present. The types of pains include sensations of **stabbing, cramping, aches (dull to severe), shooting pains** and pain that's dependant on the position of the body and the accompanying state of breathing.

Unfortunately, the pains are often mistaken for something worse than they actually are, and because they can vary in terms of the type of pain - the location on the chest and the time of day they can strike - they can often cause the anxiety victim to assume the worst about them. For example: a stabbing pain across the chest is assumed to be a heart attack, an ache is automatically acute angina and chest pressure suddenly becomes a lung problem.

Chest pains often act as the trigger for setting off **panic attacks** too - particularly when they occur alongside a heart palpitation (although they are usually mutually exclusive).

Why? There are several reasons why chest pains occur as a result of an anxiety problem. The first and primarily the most common reason is **muscle tension**. Anxiety and adrenaline cause our muscles to tense up - even when we think we're not tense - and a lot of the tension centres itself upon specific points of the body. These areas are mainly the chest, back, shoulders and abdomen.

When we're dealing with a lot of adrenaline, our muscles tense up to provide an outlet for it all. Our core upper torso muscles seem to 'scrunch up' like a sponge - acting as the body's way of dealing with the adrenaline. As a result, all sorts of muscles are expanded and contracted as a result, almost entirely against our will. Throughout the day our muscles can do this - they can happen throughout the day: at work, during chores and on social occasions.

The muscle tensing process is harmless in the long term, however in the short term all the scrunching, tensing and contracting will cause all sorts of pain that can differ from muscle to muscle. Good posture and muscle stretching is the key to alleviating the pain that tension causes, as well as taking any irrational focus away from the pain being something serious and unlikely.

Chest pains are also commonly linked with **Irritable Bowel Syndrome, indigestion** and **excess stomach gases**. Our digestion cycle can be affected by anxiety, due to our body focusing on dealing with the adrenaline and other bodily chemicals that are released during periods of high anxiety. The stomach can often produce excessive acid and gases which push up against the chest causing pressure against the sternum and chest muscles. An observation of the digestive cycle is usually required to identify this as the cause, as well as noting what you've eaten prior to chest pains occurring.

2.6 Hypersensitivity / body checking

What? During periods of anxiety we may become prone to scanning our bodies for signs of an anomaly or trying to find something that's wrong.

When we become confused about the way we feel - particularly when anxiety and panic strike unexpectedly - we can immediately turn the attention inwards on ourselves to find the cause or reasoning as to why we feel so differently.

Hypersensitivity is when we find ourselves in a state of self-observation; we are scanning our bodies to try and find problems to *justify* the intense feeling of fear we are experiencing. For example, we may think that an odd pain we experience is a sign of something serious, perhaps we become irrationally fearful of something in our environment, or a sense of *derealization* indicates that we're potentially going insane.

Unfortunately, hypersensitivity seems to work hand in hand with anxiety. When we are anxious and dealing with lots of adrenaline we may - without even acknowledging it - attach odd reasoning to why we feel the way we do. For example, when we are anxious our breathing alters (shortness of breath) and our heart often palpitates. Our reasoning may tell us that the shortness of breath and the rapid heart beat are the culprits for this anxiety, when in fact it is quite the opposite.

If you find yourself constantly scanning your body then I'm afraid that you're already anxious! It is common for most people to experience palpitations and differences in breathing that often pass unnoticed. However, when we are hypersensitive, we often 'clock on' to every twinge and difference we spot within us which just adds to the pile of worry. The breathing becomes a serious issue and the heart palpitation is suddenly something severe.

Why? Hypersensitivity occurs as a direct result of adrenaline being released into the system but, crucially, it is intensified through repetitive habit. When our body activates our **'fight or flight'** response, we immediately enter a mode of **hyperawareness** – something that's handy in times of danger and is part of our genetic makeup. However, when an anxious episode strikes, the same process happens, except that confusion often follows because there is no identifiable cause/danger in front of us. The hyperawareness can then become channeled into **hypersensitivity** and we begin to analyse ourselves.

After all, if there's no danger in front of us, or an easy explanation, then it must be our bodies that are the cause of the problem...

Over time, self-analysing or body checking can turn into a bad habit. We begin to search for things that simply are not there. The simple process of body checking causes a lot of unnecessary stress for the body to handle.

2.7 Panic attacks

What? A panic attack is when an intense feeling of fear, dread, loss of control and entrapment overwhelm a person. Accompanying these feelings are thoughts of imminent disaster, impending doom and even the fear of sudden death. A panic attack is often unexplainable and can appear to strike without an identifiable trigger. The physical symptoms that can occur alongside this are feelings of **detachment, vertigo, dizziness, light-headedness, shortness of breath, muscular pain** and various vision impairments. Panic attacks can occur infrequently (once in a while) or several times a day.

Panic attacks are often responsible for 'unnecessary' trips to the hospital and can often 'mask' themselves as a heart attack, stroke or mental 'breakdown'. The most prominent effect of a panic attack is its incredible ability to make somebody believe the most irrational and unlikeliest of scenarios and outcomes. These scenarios include the belief of sudden death against all logic (I'm having a heart attack!), the unlikely 'diagnosis' of a symptom, or the feeling that all existence will end almost immediately. Sufferers can often find the experience so terrifying that they fear it will happen again. This leads to many being stuck in the 'loop of peaking anxiety' which was mentioned in Part 1.

Why? A panic attack happens when the body releases a large amount of unexpected adrenaline into the bloodstream. Adrenaline can cause all sorts of changes both physically and mentally – the most prominent change being the stimulation of our nervous system.

If we're unprepared or 'caught off-guard' by a newly-released dump of adrenaline, then it could be expected of us to panic about this sudden change. The panic comes from the confusion over what is happening, alongside the belief that you cannot cope. Adrenaline actually causes our minds to race and be filled with all sorts of thoughts and conclusions as to *why* we're panicking and *why* we're feeling strange.

This would explain why so many people are convinced that they're having a heart attack, or that they're going insane, or that they have an incurable condition and so on. It is the adrenaline that affects our rationality during these periods of panic, thus causing them to turn into prolonged *panic attacks*.

These panic attacks don't last forever because the adrenal gland finally becomes exhausted and cannot release any further adrenaline. Our nervous systems also settle in due time. The reader should take comfort in the fact that a panic attack cannot last forever because of this, and that therefore the feeling of normality will return. It's what you do next that determines the severity, intensity and frequency of any potential panic attacks in the future.

2.8 Fear of having a panic attack

What? Fearing a panic attack itself is perhaps a clearer symptom of anxiety than any other. Many who have experienced the horrendous experience of a panic attack are in fact so terrified of one happening again that they spend the majority of their time anticipating another one. This is called being left in a state of apprehension - similar to what I explained when discussing heart palpitations above. It's actually a simplistic loop that many people have experienced or have become stuck in. This state is often exclusive to people who have been diagnosed with panic disorder.

Why? The experience of having a panic attack is often a terrifying ordeal for the individual who lives through it. Anyone who's experienced a panic attack would obviously wish to never have one again, but for some people the fear is so prominent that they spend the majority of their time self-analysing so as to apprehend one if it strikes.

The process of doing this is self-destructive as it adds to a person's overall anxiety and creates a stress that hinders daily life. Ultimately, a panic attack is a temporary loss of control and it's this loss of control that drives us to try and control every aspect of anxious thoughts and behaviours.

2.9 Nausea (feeling sick) / frequent urination / diarrhoea

What? Nausea is the feeling where it feels like we need to be sick. Frequent urination usually coincides with the need to empty our bowels on a frequent basis. Basically, we feel we need to go to the toilet a lot. Stools are found to have a liquid consistency and we may pass wind more frequently than usual.

Why? It's common knowledge that when we're anxious or nervous about something, we often feel 'woozy' or that we may be sick. Perhaps this could happen before a job interview, a public event or while awaiting important news about something. Alongside this we may find ourselves going to the toilet a lot more than usual.

Basically, all that's happening is an offshoot of the body's 'fight or flight' response. When the body prepares itself for imminent danger, it tries to relieve pressure on the organs by releasing things inside the body such as water, food, gases and stomach acid. The brain tries to pressure the stomach into pushing out all of the digesting food, acid and gases. Our bowels are rushed into action to empty everything it contains - that's why we often get diarrhoea or poor quality stools. Furthermore, the bladder begins to work overtime to try to rid the body of any excess water.

2.10 Fear of sudden death

What? This is the feeling of imminent disaster or death - against all logic and rationale. This thought could stem from a panic attack or feeling overwhelmed.

Why? When anxiety is high, so are our levels of adrenaline. High amounts of adrenaline place us firmly in 'fight or flight' mode, which alters the way we view our surroundings and prepares us for worst case scenarios. Death is arguably the foundation of any worst-case scenario, so it's not surprising that many with anxiety feel extra-sensitive when it comes to mortality. Death is *the* worst-case scenario and sometimes appears wrongly as the most obvious companion to a very intense bout of anxiety and panic.

2.11 Headaches

What? Obviously most of us will know of and have experienced many headaches in our lifetime. However, it is important to be aware that headaches come in many forms and for a variety of different reasons - this is particularly important when relating headaches to anxiety.

A headache can present itself as a <u>mild to severe aching</u> sensation, <u>short stabbing pains</u> across the scalp and temple, a <u>stretching/throbbing</u> sensation across the head and pain that seems to <u>emanate from beneath the skull</u>. The duration of a headache can vary as well, with some headaches merely spanning an afternoon, while others last for two weeks plus (my longest headache lasted over a month). The headaches can present as constant, they can alter in severity, they can 'come and go' and they can vary in their response to painkillers.

Why? Headaches can arise because of factors such as dehydration, eye strain, malnutrition, sun stroke, stress and as a symptom of another illness such as hay fever or the common cold. These name just some of the many reasons why headaches can occur. In relation to anxiety, headaches mainly occur because of <u>stress</u>, **muscle tension** and **poor posture**. Stress causes our bodies to seize up and adrenaline causes our muscles to tense up. We often and quite unknowingly alter our posture to accommodate for all of this muscle tension.

Over time poor posture - whether standing or sitting - causes the muscles on our scalp, neck and shoulders to become weathered and stretched. Our muscles are expanding and contracting all the time and the added effort of stretching *against* our poor posture causes aches and pains all over the head area. Imagine your scalp and shoulders being made of thin rubber and that rubber stretching as your posture curves inwards. Stretching and posture alteration is the key to alleviating head pains caused by muscle tension.

Dehydration and poor appetite are also contributing factors to a headache. The body cries out for nutrients and water and when this need isn't met it causes a stress on the body – this can cause a headache. Furthermore, a lack of sleep (insomnia) and a poor sleeping pattern can easily cause headaches, especially when we find ourselves overly tired.

2.12 Agoraphobia - 'the fear of going outside'

What? It is very common for a lot of people with an anxiety problem to fear going outside. Agoraphobia is, more often than not, found to be directly linked to an anxiety problem due to the irrational nature of the fear itself. To the agoraphobic person, the outside world becomes 'out of bounds', due to it being perceived as too open, too dangerous, so that they believe they **may not cope** if taken away from their current surroundings or fear how the general public may perceive them.

When I was dealing with the peak of my anxiety, I recall hardly ever leaving the house for the fear that I may have **a panic attack,** or that I simply would not cope. I also feared what my local community would think of me, which only intensified my underlying **fear of going insane**.

Why? Agoraphobia is the result of anxiety and all of the symptoms and thought associations that come with it. **Racing thoughts, unexplainable fear, irrational thinking** and **hypersensitivity** can make you perceive the world as an overwhelming place, when in fact it is the combination of your body's chemical imbalance (adrenaline) and the irrational associations and beliefs that you hold about the world outside that are overwhelming you.

Some people - particularly those who *suffer* from agoraphobia - believe that it is the outside world that's responsible for their anxious thoughts and not the other way around. This is simply not the case. We as anxiety sufferers can become agoraphobic due to the power of association we place on our surroundings, especially when anxiety is at its highest - and we feel safest in our own homes. What you must realise is that anxiety prevents you from thinking rationally, so it comes down to willpower to convince yourself that the outside world is no less of a safe place than the inside of the home.

2.13 Irritable bowel syndrome (I.B.S)

What? Irritable Bowel Syndrome (also known as spastic colon) is surprisingly common in people who have experienced a prolonged anxiety problem. Symptoms of I.B.S include **stomach bloating, acid reflux, trapped wind, constipation, diarrhoea, stomach pains, sore rectum** and **gastrointestinal discomfort**. It can also cause notable variations in the types of bowel movements that we have and the frequency with which they occur. Some people can observe which foods tend to 'trigger' the I.B.S, with some of the most common being foods that contain spice, gluten, wheat, lactose, fat and high amounts of sugar (it varies for each individual). It is not uncommon for people who have undergone large amounts of stress to develop intolerances to the foods listed above.

Why? Anxiety affects the body's chemistry, which in turn affects things such as the immune system, hormone production and the digestive cycle. I don't know the full biological process of how anxiety affects the digestive tract, but there is official medical research confirming the direct link between the two. What is known is that anxiety can cause changes to our **blood pressure, metabolism** and also create excessive amounts of **muscle tension** - particularly in the abdomen. This leaves no doubt as to the impact anxiety can have on the abdominal area, which contains the fuelling engine for our bodies.

2.14 Abdominal pains

What? Abdominal pains are those that occur across the abdomen and can vary in the way that they present. These include **feeling sore, stretching sensations, stabbing, shooting pains, cramping** and **general aching**. The location of these pains can alter in their position on the abdomen and can also fluctuate in their intensity. It is possible for a lot of these pains to coincide and to happen at any time of the day.

Why? There are two common reasons why abdominal pains can occur as a result of anxiety: the first being that the pain is an offshoot symptom of **Irritable Bowel Syndrome** (as explained above). The second, and perhaps the most common, reason is down to muscle tension and posture. Muscle tension is responsible for all types of pains due to anxiety causing us to expand and contract our muscles intensely and excessively. Adrenaline causes our muscles to tense up - even against our will - so if we don't stretch and relax accordingly, we feel the consequences through erratic and varied pain. Poor posture also intensifies this muscle tension, especially when we are hunched up and our shoulders are too far forward. Stretching, posture change and movement are the key to alleviating the pains.

2.15 Tiredness / lethargy / exhaustion

What? This is the feeling of being overly tired or lethargic in a way that ill suits the time of day. Furthermore, you could be experiencing frequent states of exhaustion that have just taken up a regular role in your day to day life.

Why? Simply living with an anxiety condition is tiring enough, as it causes the body to work hard all of the time. Anxiety can cause the body to do all sorts of 'unnecessary' overtime in the form of maintaining **a fast heart rate, taking in too much oxygen**, a **distorted digestive cycle, muscle tension**, processing **racing thoughts**, dealing with copious amounts of adrenaline and so on. Furthermore, anxiety affects sleeping patterns and the overall quality of sleep, which over time accumulates and presents itself in the form of chronic lethargy. Although troubling, tiredness is not a cause for concern and unfortunately is inevitable when anxiety is a constant.

2.16 Excessive perspiration (sweating)

What? Sweating is a normal bodily function that's intended to cool us down when our body temperature is high. However, when it becomes excessive, or occurs more frequently than usual, it usually has a direct link to anxiety. Sweating can occur when we are anxious, after strenuous exercise, after eating certain foods or whilst we are in a hot climate. It can also occur for no apparent reason - this is usually exclusive to the anxiety sufferer.

Why? When we are anxious our body temperature naturally rises due to the heart and body having to work harder. Furthermore, anxiety is also the trigger of the 'fight or flight' response and during this the body tries to push out any excess fluids through urination and sweating. When anxiety becomes a prominent feature in our lives, so do the symptoms that can occur with it - excessive perspiration being one of them. Drinking lots of water and working on the core of the problem is the solution to this.

2.17 Muscle pains & spasms

What? Muscle pains and spasms can occur all over the body, but are particularly prominent in the **chest, abdomen, back** and **shoulder** areas. A spasm is the sensation of a muscle quickly tensing and expanding against our will and can occur with or without pain. Odd twinges and pains can occur in our muscles too and they can happen in almost any muscle in our bodies.

Why? As explained before, anxiety and adrenaline cause muscle tension all over the body, which is adjunct to the body's 'fight or flight' response. It is a perfectly normal bodily reaction, but over time the constant tensing of muscles can take its toll, with the muscles becoming overly strained, inflamed and overused.

Muscle spasms are also linked to dehydration and a poor diet. Spasms and pains are very common in the chest and abdominal areas and are often mistaken for something worse. The chest, abdomen and shoulders often take most of the tension, thus making them prime spots for pains and spasms.

2.18 Dehydration / dry mouth / feeling thirsty

What? Dehydration occurs when the normal water content of your body is reduced due to releasing more water than is being taken in. Symptoms of this can include: **experiencing dry mouth, feeling thirsty, feeling lightheaded, dry lips, nausea, lethargy** and **passing urine** less frequently or in lesser amounts. Dehydration can also lead to feeling unusual or **detached from our surroundings (derealisation)**. Dehydration can also trigger **panic attacks** as it **raises the heart rate** and can make us feel **dizzy** and unstable.

Why? A water imbalance (dehydration) can occur due to a poor appetite and bad habits, where we don't take in enough water, we **excessively perspire, frequently urinate, alter our breathing** and **pass watery stools**. When we are anxious, we actually need a lot more water than usual to compensate for the loss of water.

Dry mouth can be recurrent due not only to a water imbalance, but to nasal obstruction and excess stomach acid. Stomach acid has a low PH and kills off some of the bacteria in our mouths that keep our mouth hydrated and healthy. Drinking lots of water and a healthy diet are key to alleviating dehydration and dry mouth.

2.19 Eye floaters

What? Eye floaters present themselves as strange 'blobs' or cell-like shapes that float across the eye-line regardless of where we are looking. They are small pieces of debris that can vary in size and can look like black shadowy dots, fluffy dots, long narrow strands and noose-like cells. These 'floaters' get their name because they float around the eye's vitreous humour - a jelly-like substance within the eye ball.

Why? Floaters are very common in a lot of people and are usually not the sign of a serious eye condition. They can also be the shadows that the aforementioned 'debris' casts onto the retina. In relation to anxiety, it is unknown if there is a direct link between eye floaters and anxiety.

What is known is that anxiety causes victims to be **hyperaware** and **hypersensitive** of themselves and their surroundings. Eye floaters usually pass unnoticed by many or aren't regarded to be dangerous, however, when we are anxious we can often fixate ourselves on the floaters and assume the worst about their presence.

If they do become excessive it would be wise to seek a doctor's or optician's opinion, but in most cases they are harmless. I still have the floaters in my eyes but they pass unnoticed unless I feel anxious. Anxiety causes **our peripheral vision to shut down** and our vision **to alter its focus** thus making the floaters more apparent.

2.20 Difficulty relaxing / inability to keep still

What? Anxiety often acts as a stumbling block when it comes to relaxing or trying to 'wind down'. It can cause the simplest of relaxed activities to become laboured and effortful. Activities such as reading, watching television, writing, knitting etc, can feel strenuous and unnatural.

We often worry when we aren't able to enjoy the things we usually enjoy, which can add to the overall anxiety. Moreover, a lot of activities and chores require focus and the ability to remain still. Anxiety can cause us to worry to the point where we fidget, or even pace the room in a desperate attempt to provide an outlet or to 'keep it together'.

Why? It's very difficult to relax and focus when we are anxious because of the chemical imbalance within our bodies. Adrenaline causes us to be 'on edge' as part of the body's 'fight or flight' response. It causes our minds to be flooded with copious amounts of thoughts, as well as causing physical changes to how we operate. The 'fight or flight' response is designed as a defence mechanism for when we sense danger. Unfortunately, an anxiety condition can confuse the brain when it comes to defining literal danger and imagined danger. It becomes very difficult to relax or 'switch off' as the chemicals in our body are prepared for danger instead of allowing us to relax.

2.21 Rib pains / pressure under the ribs

What? Anxiety can often be the cause for rib pains and pressure under the rib cage area. The pains can vary and can present themselves as a dull ache, sharp pains, pain in the muscles between each rib and general discomfort under the rib area. Like many other symptoms, rib pain is often misconceived as something worse than it actually is.

Why? There are two main causes for rib pain in relation to anxiety. The first is **muscle tension** and the effects of consistent muscle contraction and poor posture. The top of the abdomen, including the rib muscles, is a prime spot for muscle tension caused by anxiety. Furthermore, anxiety causes our posture to change and we can often hunch up and push our shoulders forward, which intensifies the effect of the contracting chest and rib muscles.

The second and just as common reason can be put down to **Irritable Bowel Syndrome** and **indigestion**. Indigestion, trapped wind and a poor digestive cycle can cause excess gas and stomach acid to build up in the stomach. Gravity has little effect on gases, so they naturally rise and become trapped in areas of the stomach causing a slow build up. The top of the stomach expands to cater for the excess gas and acid, which in turn causes the stomach muscles to press against the rib cage. This is responsible for a lot of rib and chest related pain.

2.22 Search engine obsession

What? We can often turn to the internet for the answers to life's questions. We can do this by using various search engines that provide us with a list of results/answers after a quick click of a button. With regards to anxiety, unhealthy search engine use is when we obsessively trawl search engines and websites for the answer to our anxiety problems.

We can often spend hours clicking, scrolling and reading mass amounts of information that usually serves to be counterproductive when trying to alleviate stress and worry.

Why? The internet has rapidly become the first and fastest point of reference for obtaining information. When we feel anxious or panicky, we often want a quick solution or fix to the problem. Unfortunately, we can often fall victim to believing that search engines have the immediate answer.

Search engines are designed to list websites that are 'best tailored' to the search that you requested. This is defined by how popular a website is, the information contained within the website or how much a web developer has paid to place their website high on the search ranking list. This leads to all sorts of websites being thrown up by search engines. It can often be hard to define which websites are set up with good intentions and which are set up solely for profit.

I would personally advise anyone to limit their internet searching, as too much information can become overwhelming and an anxious mind is susceptible to the negatives that such information might provide. Anxiety causes us to reach irrational conclusions and I have found that relating to the 'medical' research we find on sleek, professional websites does more bad than good. Go to your General Practitioner for a diagnosis.

2.23 Ringing in the ears / tinnitus

What? Tinnitus presents as a constant or broken up ringing in the ears. It can vary in pitch, volume, frequency and can often still be heard when the ears are covered. It is known to cause discomfort, **insomnia, dizziness, lightheadedness** and **panic**.

Why? Tinnitus can often be permanent as a result of damage to the internal ear. However, with regards to anxiety, I have found that tinnitus has not remained permanent with those who have managed to battle and overcome their anxiety.

There are many factors that cause tinnitus, with anxiety being a major cause. If you're experiencing it don't panic. Instead, just focus on managing your anxious thoughts and the symptoms will subside. Please visit your doctor if you have any concerns.

PART 3

NOW THAT WE'VE COVERED the 'ins and outs' of anxiety and the array of symptoms that accompany it, we can move on to making the next positive steps to actually overcoming it - just like I did many moons ago. You may or may not realise this, but just by reading up to this point of the book you have already taken a giant step towards a 'recovery', even if it doesn't feel like it yet.

The core foundation when tackling anxiety, and perhaps when dealing with almost any difficult problem in life, is to form a strong understanding of it. When we simplify a problem, it inevitably becomes easier to tackle and eventually fades to the point where it isn't actually deemed a problem at all. When we *understand* that anxiety isn't this dangerous and complex condition we initially perceived it to be, we can begin to strip it down, piece by piece, until its true harmless face is revealed.

This part of the book will provide straight up advice and steps as to what to do next to ease the persistent fear that anxiety causes and facilitate a return to normality. Remember that you're not isolated with this problem. It's alarmingly common. Even when the strangest of things happen and you're stuck in a bit of a strange place, always remember that the feelings will eventually subside and that you will return to normality.

3.1 It's just anxiety

Stop trying to work your feelings out!

Seriously, just stop. As anxiety sufferers we often become worried, confused and frustrated at the continuous and sometimes unrelenting nature of our condition. As we have learnt, the very process of worrying about our condition, as well as trying to 'work it out', only brings negative attention to the problem and acts in a way that's counterproductive when trying to alleviate all of our problems.

Just merely thinking about anxiety produces a negative effect on the mind and body. It releases adrenaline and sets us off on the same negative thought paths where we can find ourselves back at square one - worrying about why we feel the way we do and scanning ourselves for signs of disaster.

Many of us - including myself - find ourselves stuck in the same repetitive thought patterns, and in a lot of cases look for that miraculous thought/epiphany where we might feel that one thought can conquer all of our worries and symptoms. Unfortunately, this 'miracle thought' is impossible to find, as anxiety is the result of poor routine and a biological imbalance within the body. I'm sorry to say this but one thought cannot fix your problems and the only way out of a problem caused by poor routine is to trade it in for a fresh, healthier routine and a positive mental outlook.

Now this may seem easier said than done - particularly when anxiety appears to cripple us and any task seems like a physical and emotional mountain to climb. I used to think simple tasks such as posting a letter or going to the shops was out of my reach. It's also common thinking that the prospects of change, doing something different or taking ourselves out of our comfort zones, is an action that will set us up for a fall. Thoughts revolving around negative outcomes like 'not being able to cope' and fearing panic attacks often act as stumbling blocks to actually getting out and establishing a new routine.

In order to take your second step towards overcoming anxiety (the first being the establishment of your understanding), you need to **immediately implement a change in your behavioural patterns**. Stop trying to work it out because, quite frankly, there isn't anything to work out! You know what anxiety is, where it has come from and what happens within your body when anxiety and panic strike. You need to snap out of a routine that is only promoting anxiety and irrational thinking and start a new one. It is a scary prospect but it doesn't take long for your positive actions to quell the severity of your scary thoughts.

Now you may be questioning why and how this would help at all. Let me explain using a common scenario:

"Rebecca has been suffering with generalised anxiety and panic disorder for around three years. She finds it very difficult to leave the house and as a result of this lost her job a year ago. She lives on her own and hasn't the confidence to get back in touch with her friends, or establish new relationships due to fear of leaving the house and struggling with severe social anxiety. She wishes she could feel like she 'used to', or return to a time from *before* the anxiety started.

Almost every day she wakes up hoping to feel 'normal' again but is immediately disappointed when she finds that she still feels the same and that there are still odd things happening to her body. Her first thought when she wakes up is *'Do I feel okay today?'*. When she doesn't feel the way she wants to, she starts to panic. She panics because yet again everything doesn't feel normal and that she feels like she's living with an incurable, psychological condition. The panic then defines the world around her and sways any decisions and motivation that could have existed with the freshness of waking up from sleep.

Her thoughts then turn on herself. She begins to body scan. *'Why have I still got this headache?'*, *'this pain is still here'*, *'something is seriously wrong with me'*, *'I feel like I'm going insane!'* she often thinks. She then starts to try and rationalize and apply logic to give herself hope: *'I'll work this out! It'll be something deep and complex but once I've found the answer I'll be okay again!'*

Rebecca proceeds to pace around her house and exhaust herself. Every day she waits for the feelings to pass, or for that miracle thought to enter her head. Sometimes, when she feels okay, she reasons with herself that the anxiety has passed. This is until the symptoms of anxiety crop up again. Her chest flutters, she feels lightheaded, her breathing changes and her mind is flooded with undesirable thoughts. She's back to square one. *'What's wrong with me?'"*

It's obvious from this scenario that Rebecca has been confined to her own negative thought patterns and has fallen victim to abiding by her own sense of irrationality. Rebecca is constantly anxious and has found herself stuck in the 'loop of peaking anxiety'. Rebecca believes that her problems will go away through her abiding by the same anxiety-dictated routine and thought patterns that revolve around worry. She thinks that simply by waiting and trying to 'think her way out' of it she will eventually get to where she wants. As the case study said, she has been suffering for three years.

What Rebecca needs to do – and this applies to all of us - is to change her behaviours, both physical and mental, from the moment she wakes up. She needs to realise that there is nothing to work out - she simply has anxiety. Instead of waking up and thinking *'Am I okay today?'*, she needs to think, *'Okay, well I've had anxiety and these symptoms for a while now. I accept this and I'm going to do something productive today regardless of how I feel'.*

We need to realise that our bodies take time to recover from the symptoms anxiety can produce. Pains, aches, derealisation, an imbalance of adrenaline and all of the other symptoms can take a while to subside, but they *will* subside given the chance. So for now just ignore them. Rebecca needs to ignore how she feels because she *knows* she has anxiety and a plethora of things 'wrong' with her.

With that out of the way, we can now begin to change our behavioural habits. Positive rationalisation tells us that the outside is no more of a danger than sitting inside. Setting goals that challenge our fears, such as going outside, begins the process of rewiring the default thought process of our brains.

The more we rely on emotional crutches, such as the walls of our homes, then the more we'll end up back at the beginning. The more we keep our minds occupied on tasks, hobbies, fun activities and socialising, then the less we keep our minds on bad thought patterns, such as dwelling on the anxiety or working out our problems. Believe me this works.

Set yourself a goal no matter how simple it may seem. If *you* find it a scary and difficult task then I suggest you bravely undertake it. For me it was doing the simple things like catching the bus to work, going to the supermarket or going for a short walk. You'll find that nothing bad happens despite your feelings telling you otherwise. You have to ignore your gut on this one and rely on willpower. There's no use sitting in, thinking away your problems.

This is the first step: stop working it out. In Part 1 we discussed grouping all of our symptoms and problems into one manageable problem. Using the anxiety umbrella, we can put all of our excessive and irrational worries to one side and concentrate on dealing with them as one manageable problem. This includes psychological worries about our mental health, as well as the physical worries that come with anxiety, such as derealisation, heart palpitations, chest pains, tiredness, headaches, panic attacks etc. Excessive worry is just anxiety. That's it.

Lose the *'What If?'* because it's just anxiety

It's a normal part of the human thinking process to contemplate different types of outcomes to any given situation. In *Rationality and Worst-Case Scenarios* we covered several types of irrational conclusions that our mind can lead us to when we're in a state of anxiety. What we have learned is that anxiety causes us to distort our thinking to the point where we simply focus on the frightening possibilities and less on the harmless, more likely outcomes.

As you'll know, these frightening possibilities - that manifest themselves as thoughts - can easily be dwelt upon and can often dictate our plans and actions in our daily lives. Anxiety almost always stops us from what we want to do or 'used to do' - making it a crippling stumbling block when it comes to living the life that we want to.

Both consciously and subconsciously, a life consumed by anxiety can lead us to question situations with the constant qualifying question

'*What if?*'. Applying the '*What if?*' question to scenarios in life isn't always a bad thing, with it being vital in terms of keeping us safe and avoiding any potential, negative ramifications in a given situation. When '*What If?*' is applied to justify irrational fears however, then it becomes a problem.

We can apply '*What If?*' in common situations such as approaching a blind bend when driving, choosing between walking home through a badly-lit or well-lit area or perhaps thinking twice about bringing up a sensitive topic of conversation in a group of people. This use of logic can help keep us safe and avoid any upsetting consequences that could occur, such as avoiding a car crash or offending somebody for example.

However, excessive anxiety, which often leads to hypersensitivity and hyperawareness, can create an abundance of '*What if?*' in our lives, which can lead us to apply the question to normal every day things. We can start to question our normal daily actions and the '*What if?*' starts to take centre-stage when we begin to apply our logic. Normal every day activities, such as going outside, going to social occasions or even taking the journey to work, can suddenly be perceived as dangerous tasks that would be best left avoided, due to fear of a panic attack or something awful happening.

Furthermore, from a hypochondriac perspective, we can also begin to question the symptoms that occur with anxiety. We can begin to look at feeling different, experiencing bodily changes and all of the other symptoms that come with anxiety as something that's a 'worst-case scenario'. For example: a headache becomes a brain tumour, a palpitation becomes a heart defect, or a sense of derealisation is the first sign of insanity.

Let us look at some rational and irrational *What If's* to clarify.

Rational 'What If' Scenarios

- *"I really want to stay for another drink"* - What if I'm too drunk to get up for work?
- *"I can't be bothered to go back for my bike helmet"* - What if I have an accident?
- *"I'll risk not wearing a jacket today"* - What if it rains?
- *"I want to make a joke about this subject"* - What if I offend my colleague?
- *"I think that stray dog looks friendly"* - What if it suddenly attacks?

Irrational 'What If' Scenarios

- *"I need to go and get the grocery shopping"* - What if something bad happens outside?
- *"I must get the busy train to work"* - What if I have a panic attack?
- *"My heart keeps pounding and skipping beats"* - What if I have a heart attack?
- *"My friend has invited me to a party"* - What if they think badly of me?
- *"Everything suddenly feels different"* - What if I'm going insane?
- *"The doctor says there's nothing wrong with me"* - What if I've been misdiagnosed?

We all use irrationality to shape and strengthen our use of rational thinking and logic. Therefore, ironically, the process of irrational thinking is in actual fact a *rational* process. It only becomes a problem when the irrational thought becomes our conclusion - a walk to the shops becomes categorically too dangerous, for example.

This is where the next and arguably most difficult step arises in overcoming anxiety. **You have to lose the *'What if?'*.** In order to lose it, you first need to do something that sounds simple, but actually takes a lot of willpower to apply. You need to identify the irrational *'What if?'* and simply ignore it. In order to identify and ignore it, you need to dig deep and use your own sense of positive rationalisation and apply it to the scenarios where you think anxiety is stopping you from doing the things you should, or need to, be doing.

When I was struggling at the peak of my anxiety, I wouldn't even leave the house. I feared what the outside world would think of me if I suddenly became overwhelmed with anxiety or had a panic attack. One day I decided to lose the *'What if?'* and actually used positive logic to weigh up the possible outcomes of leaving the house. I decided I needed to go food shopping and in doing so ignored all the feelings, thoughts and emotions I was going through in order to do it.

I managed to make it to the supermarket and almost had a panic attack in the vegetable aisle. I was so close to turning around and running home, but I stuck at it and *imagined* the pride I'd feel if I completed the shopping. I did eventually complete the shopping and the sense of achievement I felt when I got home actually helped ease the anxiety I was feeling. I was scared of the *possibility* of something bad happening, not the *reality*. I also realised that my home was my 'safe place' and that I was using it as an emotional crutch. Going to the supermarket helped me to temporarily live without this.

Positive rationalisation is a fancy-named term that's the equivalent of saying *'It's just anxiety'* out loud. Lose the *'What if?'* and blame everything that scares you on anxiety. Pop up your anxiety umbrellas and let them shield you from the monsoon of irrationality that rains upon you. Get out there and have a go!

It really is 'just anxiety'

In section 1.1 we looked at grouping all of the thoughts, fears and symptoms together. We labeled them as one problem and I explained about the use of the *Anxiety Umbrella*. A good way to distinguish between a 'normal' symptom and a symptom of anxiety, is to look at it comparatively with a time where you once felt okay. What also helps is that sometimes, deep down, we know that our thinking can become quite absurd, so we can use positive rationalisation to identify what thoughts are normal and what thoughts are caused by the anxiety.

I cannot stress enough the benefits of labeling our symptoms and fears as 'anxiety'. We know that anxiety will eventually ease and what helps is that an onslaught of several symptoms at one time can be found to be manageable, with the knowledge that they're only caused by one thing! For example, you could be suffering from a prolonged headache, experiencing a lack of appetite, worrying about chest pains and perhaps being scared to attend a social event. These are several different symptoms to contend with, but they don't need to be dealt with individually. **They are all just anxiety**. They will all pass in due time and if they don't go away then you're more than likely refusing to accept that it's just anxiety.

On the next page is a diagram consisting of common symptoms where anxiety is directly involved:

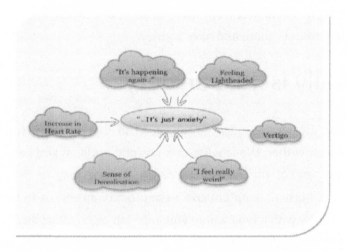

As you can see from the example above, there are several listed anxiety symptoms which all point to one common cause - anxiety itself. Each symptom on its own can be found to be scary or discomforting and it doesn't take a lot for the anxiety sufferer to imagine how overwhelming it feels for these symptoms to be happening all at once. Anxiety can be blamed for many other feelings and symptoms - most of which are listed in **Part 2**of this book. Let us look at another example:

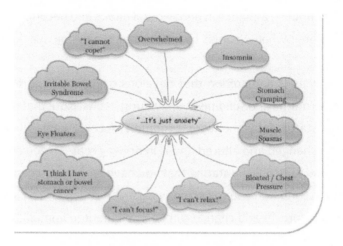

As you can see in scenario 2, there seem to be several symptoms happening at the same time, but they are all linked to one cause. I and many others have found that we've had many more symptoms happening at once or recurring frequently. The only thing that linked them all was anxiety. Anxiety creates so much stress on the body and we must realise that the symptoms can come in abundance. Put it all down to anxiety and you'll quickly find that it becomes a manageable problem to contend with.

There's nothing 'wrong' with you

Suffering with anxiety, regardless of how long you have put up with the condition, should not be feared as there isn't actually anything wrong with you. This is arguably a bold statement to announce, given all the turmoil and emotional distress anxiety can cause. However, a major key to recovery is to realise that anxiety itself is not an illness; it is definitely not dangerous and can be fixed through the uses of a strong understanding, a change in behavioural habits and becoming a reflective practitioner when it comes to tracking and analysing our thoughts.

Anxiety is a condition that develops over time as a result of poor mental routine and solidified behavioural habits. Note that the key word in that statement is the word 'condition'. A condition is something that can be changed and altered and is in no way represented as something permanent. Simply by stating that you have an anxiety condition means that the condition you're currently in can be changed. You are not stuck with this forever and change can be implemented immediately.

Anxiety is not an illness simply because it's a bodily process that occurs naturally. Think about it; we wouldn't deem breathing, our digestive cycle, sweating and sleeping as a problem or illness - it's simply something that our body does naturally. Anxiety should be placed into the same bracket as this because all that's happening within our body is completely natural. It's an overuse of our 'fight or flight' response. We're simply dealing with the effects of living with an erratic adrenal gland and over stimulated nerves. The abnormal feelings and symptoms that come with it are merely a matter of perception. Let me explain further:

The most difficult part of dealing with the anxiety is undoubtedly the *fear* it triggers within us. We fear that of definitive change, but quite ironically most of us wish that we could change back to how we felt before the anxiety started. We've learned that the feeling of fear comes predominantly from the chemicals that are released into our bodies, mostly adrenaline and cortisol, as well as any emotional recognition attached to a given thought.

The fear - caused by this chemical imbalance - acts as the main factor when we mould our perception of the anxiety. We are quick to assume that anxiety is this terrifying and crippling burden that has been thrust upon us, instead of simply acknowledging that it's a naturally occurring bodily process that's as harmless as the hiccups or trapped wind.

As a result of habit, we consciously and subconsciously *tell* ourselves to be anxious and actually self-trigger the fight or flight response in our bodies. We fall into the same thought habits by dwelling on the same daily worries, thus giving us the same daily anxious response.

This needs to change.

It is not the fault of our adrenal gland and it is not the fault of our bodies. It is *your* thoughts that are the cause! Begin to change your thought patterns and you'll begin to change your anxiety for the better.

The power of thought

Your body reacts to all types of thoughts. Your body constantly reacts to these thoughts by releasing chemicals such as adrenaline, thus causing your body's natural balance to be constantly disturbed. Never underestimate the power of a thought and what it can do to your body!

Take a moment to think deeply about how much a thought can massively affect the body. It's something that we already know and have acknowledged on a subconscious level, but it's essential that we use this knowledge, as it acts as one of the key weapons when tackling and understanding anxiety. Let us look at a few examples:

❖ Try to think of something that excites you or remember a time where you felt overwhelmed with excitement. E.G.*a holiday, a gig, a first date, seeing a close friend, a new episode of your favourite TV program, an adventure, a hobby etc.*

It is the <u>thought</u> that excites you because you're imagining being in a desirable position. You know that you're going to enjoy the exciting event/occasion, because you've either done it previously, or are eagerly anticipating a new positive experience. Take note of the surroundings when these exciting thoughts occur.

You could be at work, walking down the street, doing the ironing or being just about anywhere. More often than not the surroundings would have little to do with you dwelling on these positive thoughts, because you're thinking about what is planned for the future (of course your surroundings can trigger the thought if it reminds you of something). Note how the body can react to what you see in your imagination, as well as what you can see in front of you.

❖ Try to think of something that scares you. E.G. *a rollercoaster, spiders, enclosed spaces, fear of losing a loved one, open water, dying.*

Even in the safe comfort of your own space, these thoughts can affect the body. When I comprehend the thought of a spider crawling across my face, scuba diving in an underwater cavern or perhaps thinking that I'm going insane, it does cause me some minor discomfort.

When dwelling on this thought I can safely say that I'd be in no mood to engage in one of life's laborious activities. What about those feelings of dread before a job interview? Or an upcoming meeting with somebody or something that frightens you? Once again these thoughts can have little to do with what's around you, with only your surroundings serving as a reminder. Simply by imagining myself in these undesirable positions has caused my body to react in its own way. Can you see what I'm puzzling together here?

The point I'm putting across is that it is _thoughts_ that can affect the body. Anxious thoughts are part of being human, but excessive worry and negative thoughts can and _will_ affect the balance of the body. When anxiety is largely understood this imbalance is easily rectified, however when we find ourselves in a poor mental state - crippled by fear and racing thoughts - it becomes harder to think clearly and rationally. Just say to yourself, _"I will think about this when the anxiety and the adrenaline has passed. I'm too anxious to think clearly at the moment."_

Bear this in mind the next time you find yourself dwelling on your anxiety or any scary thought. The thoughts can affect the body and it's no wonder we find ourselves in such negative states if we're constantly feeding ourselves negative thoughts. Just remember that negative thoughts create negative emotions.

We often dwell on what scares us as a way of coping with the issue, even if the event has happened or may happen in the future. It provides us with a false sense of control about an issue that scares us. Just let anxiety run its course without providing it with any more fuel. If you can achieve this then you're well on your way to beating anxiety and demonstrating a strong understanding of it.

Anxiety should not be feared

Sounding like I'm highlighting the obvious, anxiety often evokes the feeling of fear. However, anxiety itself should not be feared. If we fear anxiety and panic occurring, then we simply bring it on ourselves. Just by fearing anxiety, we evoke exactly the same emotion we feel when we are anxious! We need to <u>constantly remind ourselves that anxiety cannot hurt us</u>. Just remember that anxiety is just another name for the body's 'fight or flight' response, which is constantly irritated and triggered by worry and fear.

Let's just think about it. If a fluffy bunny rabbit came hopping towards you in the street, your body wouldn't suddenly change and release adrenaline because you do not fear it. You *know* the rabbit is coming but your body doesn't enter 'fight or flight' mode because there is no dangerous association that your mind has formed of the bunny rabbit.

Now let's switch the bunny rabbit with a rabid dog and re-run the same scenario. This time the dog comes towards us and our 'fight or flight' mode does kick in. Anxiety starts because we are worried about the danger in front of us - rapidly foraging through scenarios in our minds about what the rabid dog could do to us. This 'fight or flight' mode is there to protect us and kick start our bodies in the face of danger. Unlike the bunny rabbit, our mind associates the rabid dog as a danger.

It all boils down to perception. If you perceive feeling the symptoms of anxiety as a danger, then you'll spiral into a pit of worry that takes a long time to climb out of. Every time that you start to feel different, whether it be experiencing derealisation, obsessing on a thought or feeling something physical, then this is a time to test yourself. <u>It's all about your reaction.</u>

Treat feeling anxious as the bunny rabbit instead of the rabid dog. There's no need to add heaps of worry onto what the body is currently experiencing. The feeling will pass and will actually present itself less and less severely the more you train yourself to just tolerate it. You'll find that your anxious episodes become less frequent and also less intense. This is explained further in the following sections.

3.2 Change the bad habits. Re-wire your brain

Stop over-thinking and 'body checking'

It's ever so common for the average anxiety sufferer to over-think their problems and to try to 'think their way out of it'. We have learned that this is merely counterproductive and actually acts as a catalyst for the anxiety to kick-start. When we think about anxiety and try to 'think it away', we are actually adding another worry onto all of the other worries that we may currently be dealing with.

We also bring a large amount of attention to the anxiety which, for our hypersensitive bodies, puts us on high alert for change and danger. We don't want these anxious feelings to be present, so we're constantly on lookout for any sign of it disappearing, as well as trying to spot signs of it progressing or 'getting worse'.

Furthermore, when we are unaware or forget that anxiety has grasped hold of us, we sometimes look inwards for signs of something wrong. Many anxiety sufferers turn to scanning the body in order to attach reasoning for why they feel the way that they do. This is often the case when adrenaline is pumping through our bodies and that we have failed to acknowledge that we're currently in an anxious state.

Many people suddenly put immeasurable amounts of focus on something that they wouldn't normally deem so troublesome. This focus could be on many things, such as a change in breathing, a chest flutter, chest pains, dizziness, vertigo, derealisation, irritable bowel syndrome, ringing in the ears and so on.

What makes this deplorable is that we can cause ourselves to worry further about the symptoms we are focusing on, which in turn can cause the overall effect of the symptom to become worse or increase in intensity. For example:

Anxiety and worrying can cause heart palpitations. Worrying about the palpitations causes anxiety. With increased anxiety come more frequent palpitations, which are perceived as being 'worse', or more intense due to the extreme focus that's placed on them. You can summarise it as a two-way process. Anxiety causes palpitations. Palpitations cause anxiety. Take a look at this diagram for a clear picture:

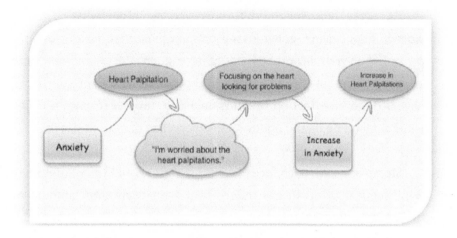

This isn't just the case for heart palpitations. Over-thinking and focusing on other symptoms unfortunately causes the same effect. For example, worrying about a headache causes stress and tension, which can actually make it worse. Worrying about chest pains causes us to tense up, causing any current chest pain to increase in intensity. Worrying about I.B.S disrupts our digestive cycle, thus making that a further problem too. This also applies to sweating, feeling sick, tinnitus, various muscle pains etc.

The very process of worrying about the anxiety actually makes the anxiety present itself with increased intensity. This is something that we have covered during the earlier stages of this book. When we over-think, or try to 'think our way out' of, anxiety we actually bring attention to the fact that it's there – affecting our lives. We become hypersensitive to it, thus making it feel more intense. The anxiety takes a more prominent presence in daily life, therefore making it feel like a bigger problem than it actually is.

Of course, worrying doesn't make every symptom worse. If you're worried about dying, going insane or something that lies out of your control, then your anxiety remains at its 'capped limit'. Remember that anxiety cannot kill you and that the thought processes of your mind have little to no effect on the outside world. Anxiety reaches a limit - with that limit being the undesirable emergence of a panic attack.

Stop placing so much focus on your symptoms and I guarantee they will disappear or drastically reduce over a relatively short amount of time. Acknowledge when they are reducing and make the link between your new thought routine and the reduction in anxiety. **Stop over-thinking and body checking**. In order to make this task easier, you need to keep your mind occupied in a healthy way.

Do what you'd usually do or try something new!

Keeping your mind occupied is undoubtedly one of the best things to do when snapping out of a bad routine crammed full of bad habits. In a lot of cases, in particular relating to my battle with anxiety, the anxiety sufferer is found to have a lot of time on their hands for aimlessly thinking about all sorts of issues and the complexities of life. Or in a lot of cases, particularly if you're a person who has a natural tendency to worry, we think about things that trouble us. We often do this because it acts as a coping mechanism in case the issues we worry about ever strike, or we treat it as a life puzzle for our minds to form an answer to.

The process of doing this isn't necessarily a bad thing. However, if we're already stuck with an anxiety condition then this 'thinking time' is often put to bad use. It's ever so common for many to use this time to dwell upon the anxiety and the symptoms that it causes. We know from the previous section, and throughout this book, that thinking and focusing attention on the anxiety is a counterproductive process. We bring attention to the issue, which actually makes it more of a problem.

Anxiety, very sadly, stops many from doing what they would usually do in their everyday lives. Activities, hobbies, socialising and daily requirements, such as work and chores, can easily become a no-go zone for many, which is why anxiety often leads to depression. Depression kills our motivation and any positive associations we have formed with what we used to deem to be fun or interesting - making it even harder for the anxiety sufferer to motivate themselves to break out of their negative routine.

This is where I lay down the next piece of advice for you and I think that it's essential that you follow it. Simply **do what you would usually do**. If you feel that the positive association you had with your old life has been all but lost then simply **try something new**. As an anxiety sufferer you need to re-wire your brain into a new, positive routine - something that does not happen overnight, but gets incredibly easier over a short amount of time.

Doing what you'd usually do doesn't mean acting out your current anxiety-fuelled routine; it means partaking in something that you once recognised as necessary for your daily life. You may have to cast your mind back way into the past for this, depending on how long you've been hampered by anxiety. This includes doing things which you once enjoyed, or just acted out without a second thought. I remember enjoying taking the busy train to the beach, filing away paper work for my job and spending time with all of my friends. These things I did without question, but became disillusioned with them during my time with anxiety.

Wake up and imagine what you would do with your day if you didn't have the anxiety - and do it anyway! The effects of a poor thought routine will try to stop you on your journey, but remember to just ignore them. Thoughts cannot harm you.

Change your reaction and you'll change the anxiety

To begin re-wiring your brain in order to cope with or rid yourself of anxiety, you'll need to change your behavioural habits. The best way to do this is to firstly monitor how you react to the dumps of adrenaline that are released into your system, or in other words, how you react to suddenly becoming overwhelmed by anxiety or panic.

When I reached a saturation point during my struggle with anxiety, I literally hit a point where I tried to not care anymore. It was a motivation dictated by anger. This was an anger deriving from the predicament I was in. I had reached 'the end of my tether' and was disgusted at how my life was being dictated to by this anxiety. I decided that I would do what I would usually do, regardless of how I felt, just to regain a sense of control in a life where I felt control was scarce.

So, I took it upon myself to live out a 'normal' daily schedule and simply use willpower to ignore any changes or symptoms that anxiety threw at me. Every time I experienced an episode of derealisation, panic, chest pains and breathlessness - I just carried on. I continued doing what I set out to do and was in no way going to let anxiety prevent me from doing it. I did the house chores, I watched a movie, I went to visit friends and I walked the dog.

Now the symptoms of anxiety did crop up, but by simply trying to ignore them and keeping my mind focused, they actually didn't feel as intense as they usually did. Be under no illusion - I still felt pretty terrible and continuously on high alert, but I did notice an incremental difference in the severity of my anxious feelings. I changed my reaction to the anxiety by simply continuing with what I was doing. My reaction changed. I was beginning to re-wire my brain.

The symptoms still felt horrible, but what I noticed was that by keeping my mind occupied and focused on something else, I only felt the anxiety at about 60% of the intensity that I had when confined to the walls of the house - focusing on my problems.

I'd caught on to something quite remarkable.

I decided to experiment with this approach, as it took the sting out of the anxious feelings I was experiencing on a daily basis. The anxiety was still there, but it didn't feel crippling anymore; it was more like a debilitating feeling that I could push through. I thought that if keeping my mind occupied helped ease the anxiety a little, then maybe it could have a cumulative effect in terms of continuously easing the anxiety. I thought that maybe the more I kept myself busy, then the less my anxiety would be present. If anxiety ever struck, then I would force my reaction to be minimal and keep my focus away from concentrating on the symptoms.

This is actually something that works so well that you can actually notice a significant difference in a matter of days. There are stages of the day where you can actually feel 'normal' and, to some degree, content with the situation.

My reaction to the anxiety was always under the spotlight.

I tried my absolute best to keep a low-level reaction when anxiety struck and, quite incredibly, I noticed the frequency and intensity of the anxious episodes slowly decrease.

You must work on your reaction to the anxiety - particularly when panic strikes. Use positive rationalisation to assume that there is nothing wrong. Just assume that it's the feeling of anxiety and continue with whatever you were doing or channel your focus onto something productive. I have worked with many people using this plan and they will tell you that this approach works. It takes time and energy but the results happen quicker than you'd think. You will surprise yourself.

Give yourself something to look forward to

Further to changing your reaction to the anxiety, you can also take a step forward by facilitating the adrenaline that pumps through your system. This book has repeatedly emphasised that adrenaline and other bodily chemicals, such as cortisol, are prime factors when it comes to the *feeling* of being anxious. However, adrenaline and fear don't always run parallel with each other. We mustn't forget that adrenaline forms a part of other positive feelings that we experience - the feeling of excitement for example.

When we feel excited, this feeling is stimulated by various chemicals – including adrenaline. Further to this, adrenaline helps us to enjoy things such as exercise, competitive activities, sport, sex, and responding to pressure. As explained before, adrenaline also forms the main part of our 'fight or flight' response, which is a vital bodily function which aids us in keeping us safe and helps us to mould our perception of what we deem safe and dangerous.

A key skill required to gain back a sense of control over your anxiety is to try and channel your thoughts down a more positive thought path. You can do this by thinking and focusing on something that you're really looking forward to and are excited at the prospect of doing. This actually helps in more ways than one, because it helps 'take the edge off' any depression (or helps prevent it) and also eases the load on the adrenal gland and nervous system.

By steering your thought path to something you can enjoy, you are channeling the adrenaline into doing something that it is useful.

Try and focus on something that actually lifts your mood. Common examples include looking forward to a holiday, attending an exciting event, a new episode of a TV show, a visit from a relative, a day out, or even 'pay day'.

Anxiety, along with depression, is often described as possessing an inability to see a positive future. By trying to focus on something that you enjoy - no matter what it is - you are actually taking a step in a positive direction - regardless of whether the enthusiasm is there or not. So, give your body a positive outlet for the adrenaline by thinking of something that's exciting or that you're looking forward to.

Don't associate feeling anxious with future events

When we think of doing anything under the influence of anxiety, our perception and emotional recognition with what we're thinking about can often become skewed. Anxiety often leads us into thinking that simple tasks are actually monumental in terms of using energy and draining us emotionally. Furthermore, when we try to think at a time when our bodies are dealing with a chemical imbalance, this can often lead us to associate the feeling of fear with activities and events that we're thinking about doing in the future.

In this part of the book I have explained that you should do what you would usually do in a situation, or try something new, as a way of breaking out of an anxious routine. I explained that this requires willpower and conjuring up the ability to ignore anxiety when it skews your thoughts and tries to distract your attention with its symptoms. When anxiety skews your thoughts, it can extinguish any enthusiasm you may have for planning positive things to do in the future. Take these common scenarios for example:

- "I'm feeling horribly anxious and I don't think I'll make the birthday party this weekend."
- "I don't want to visit the doctor. I'm going to hear something awful."
- "The last thing I want to do is go to the gym."
- "I don't think I'll cope with visiting relatives next week."
- "I'm in no state to go to work tomorrow."
- "I haven't got the energy to do the house work today."

These statements all have one thing in common. They are all a pre-emptive assumption about a future emotional state. The fact is that we don't know how we'll feel in the future, but as anxiety sufferers we have become used to the ever present, predictable nature of anxiety and the symptoms that accompany it. We unfortunately *assume* what we'll feel like in the future.

Yes, anxiety can and will drain our enthusiasm and lead us into depressive states. But the key here is to not make plans based on a current state of mind or present emotion. Yes, you'll probably be anxious at the time of making a plan, but like I explained before, you should just do it anyway. You don't know how you'll feel in a year's time, a week's time, an hour's time or even a minute's time.

By second guessing your emotional state, you're actually *choosing* what mindset to be in when the event or scenario arises. Instead of pre-empting how you'll feel, try and take a gamble and see if it pays off. Let's take those presumptions from above and re-mould them using positive rationalisation:

- "I realise that I'm anxious, but maybe the party this weekend will take my mind off of it. I may find that I actually have fun!"
- "I probably will be anxious at the doctors, but I know it's just anxiety and I'll feel better afterwards after some closure."
- "I'm unmotivated for the gym, but maybe it'll provide an outlet for all of this adrenaline."
- "I'm sure I'll be in a better mood to visit Grandma next week. I'll plan it anyway."
- "I'm anxious tonight but after some sleep I'll be alright for work. I'll do it anyway and show this anxiety no attention."
- "I can keep my mind occupied by doing some household tasks. I'm sure that when I start, I'll get into it."

Don't let a current anxious state dictate what you plan to do for the future. In fact, you shouldn't let it get in the way of what you want to do now. Use positive rationalisation and willpower and refrain from giving your anxiety any undeserved attention.

Stop researching your symptoms on the internet!

As anxiety sufferers, we can forgive ourselves for trying to find the answers to a problem that we're confused and worried about. Unfortunately, many of us turn to the internet for our answers. Quite ironically - and in contrast to one of the main ways this book can be discovered - trawling the internet usually serves to fuel anxiety and panic instead of alleviating it.

You must remember that when you type your symptoms into a search engine, you are entering data into an almost entirely pure marketspace. Almost the entire internet is a capitalist-fuelled world, where people buy and sell products, services and information. When typing anything into a search engine, you are presented with these products and services with the top search results represented by the websites who are the most popular, or who are the highest bidders. This is the same market through which I sell this book.

You'll be aware that the world around us presents us with a variety of advertising and selling techniques usually revolving around the concept of false 'need' instead of 'want'. Unfortunately, when typing health matters into a search engine, we are presented with a plethora of websites offering to sell us products, medicines, cures and methods to 'help' us with our problem. One of the most commonly used and easiest methods in marketing is the practice of 'scaremongering' people and using them as the target market.

As an anxiety sufferer, it's a very common behaviour to type our symptoms into search engines as a measure for providing relief from our panic and the feeling of being isolated. Sadly, this is where many businesses have formed a target market. We as anxiety sufferers are in need of help and many online businesses see this as an opportunity to sell their products, while the legitimacy of them is always under scrutiny.

Referring back to *Anxiety and Worst-Case Scenarios,* these websites serve to use scaremongering tactics to make us aware of these worst-case scenarios. Typing isolated common symptoms of anxiety such as palpitations, headaches, dizziness and panic, causes our screens to become flooded with cleverly, sugar-coated scaremongering techniques aimed at trying to persuade us to buy products, or scaring us into a sense of insecurity where we're at risk of purchasing something due to our state of vulnerability.

You may have found that symptoms such as heart palpitations are directly linked to a heart defect. Chest pains are almost certainly a sign of angina and chest problems. There's a good chance that your headaches are the sign of a brain tumour and dizziness is probably related to a life-threatening blood pressure problem. Although there are plausible links to these extreme cases, probability tells us they are simply the uncommon, worst-case scenario with the odds being further heightened by the fact that you have anxiety.

Furthermore, websites such as forums, blogs and chat rooms include people who thrive off of the fear they can create. Of course, I find the vast majority of forum members and bloggers are found to be perceptibly kind and helpfully-opinionated. However, when we're anxious we are easily drawn to the negative elements due to the underlying fear and adrenaline that drives us to find a solution to our problems. People can be quick to share an extreme story about someone they know or have heard about. Usually, stories that are way out of the norm draw immediate interest. This interest then represents itself in its search engine ranking.

For example, *Blogger A* writes about how a woman he once knew collapsed and died after having a headache at work. Or how *Forum Member 1* explained how his friend once had a heart palpitation leading to his heart exploding. These types of stories are prominent at the top of search engines as anything out of the norm gains large amounts of interest.

Stop using search engines to find the answers to your symptoms, unless you use a logical and rational approach. The internet isn't just filled with tripe like that mentioned above, but just be careful when differentiating between legitimate information and unethical sales pitches.

If you're looking for something then you'll find it

When we're confused about an anxious state we find ourselves in, we often look for a reason we can attach to the unexplained anxiety. We can often fall into bad habits as explained before, such as body checking, focusing on harmless symptoms, or even using our imaginations to conjure irrational dangers in our outside environment.

There are also many other things that we seem to point the finger of blame towards. Such blame can revolve around our personal and social lives, as well as us questioning our own mental health.

Anxiety sufferers - including myself at one point - often make it part of their common daily routine to knowingly or unknowingly search for blame or a reason as to why they feel the way they do. This behaviour can easily become obsessive, but often disguises itself in a normal daily routine. When we obsess, particularly when it relates to anxiety, we almost always think we have the right conclusion in our minds, but we're just searching for clarification or evidence to justify it.

For example, when we feel anxious, we can often find ourselves trying to 'think our way out of' anxiety. When this approach doesn't seem to work, we can easily conclude that something must be wrong with our mind. However, we've already had our mind made up that something is wrong, because why else would we try to think our way out of anxiety? We've already assumed that something is wrong because why would we do something so irrational as to search for a miracle thought to rid us of anxiety?

This type of obsessive thought can be applied to when we try to analyse our symptoms too. Take heart palpitations for example. If we convince ourselves that something is wrong with our heart, we can often find ourselves obsessing and focusing intensely on the rhythm and beating of the heart. Almost every person's heart beats out of a predictable rhythm at least once a day and it passes unnoticed. However, to the obsessive anxiety sufferer it becomes highly noticeable and immediately a problem. The anxiety sufferer assumes there's something wrong with the heart and so sets out to find a reason to justify the assumption. They find the reason to attach to the way they feel, without realising that all they were feeling was just anxiety.

This can be applied to many other symptoms: stomach pains, headaches, dizziness, chest pains, derealisation - to name a few. As explained in *Stop Over-Thinking and Body Checking,* this process is counterproductive and actually deflects our focus from the actual problem. In a nutshell, obsessing about something that frightens you, with regards to anxiety, means you'll more than likely find what you're looking for.

3.3 Helpful Anxiety Advice

Score your anxiety levels

When you begin to notice differences in your anxiety levels, particularly when they become less intense, you can begin to give them a rating in terms of intensity and how anxious you feel at a given time. This really helps when it comes to looking at your anxiety comparatively and you can use it to measure and acknowledge how you're progressing. It's also helpful for target setting and acts as a motivational tool to try something that we might initially feel uncomfortable with.

I began to score my anxiety when I could safely deem that the majority of my usual week felt 'normal' - where the feeling of abnormal anxiety was outweighed by the feeling of content. This is not to say that I completely rid myself of anxiety and as a matter of fact it still creeps up on me now and then - to this present day. I still use this scoring method as it acts as a reminder of how far I have come and I couldn't recommend it any more strongly than I recommend this entire book.

Turn over for the anxiety scoring method. This method can be altered and tailored for the individual. I personally use this one. Nowadays my anxiety usually averages at around a score of 2 or 3.

Anxiety Scoring Method:-

1 - 2 = Low level anxiety. No different from the average person. Usually represented by a feeling of anticipation or the feeling of impatience. Feeling stresses from a to-do list or a daily routine.

3 - 6 = Moderate Anxiety. Aware that there's a generous amount of adrenaline in the body. Feeling fairly uncomfortable and unable to relax. Intrusive thoughts and a significant effort to ignore irrational thoughts. Able to acknowledge that the feeling will pass.

7 - 9 = High Anxiety. Symptoms prominent particularly depersonalisation. Breathless and aware of symptoms such as derealisation, feelings of dread, palpitations, dizziness, vertigo and any other that has been obsessed about. Unable to think clearly or operate at a normal level both physically and emotionally. Scanning for signs of disaster. No motivation except for escape.

10 = Panic Attack. The feeling of complete derealisation, depersonalisation, confusion and imminent disaster. Panic symptoms aplenty. The feeling of no escape and impending doom. Common symptoms include a pounding chest, breathlessness, inability to focus and balance. Complete breakdown in attachment to surroundings.

The scoring method is exactly how it presents. Instead of saying to yourself, *"Oh no it's the anxiety again,"* you can actually score your anxiety and look at it comparatively. One day you may feel a bit uneasy, so instead of just folding to the assumption that it's anxiety, you could actually say to yourself, *"well I feel quite uneasy and my anxiety feels at around a 4. "*You can begin to look at anxiety as measurable.

By scoring your anxiety, you're actually establishing a preventative process where you've acknowledged how you currently feel and can immediately start to ignore certain thoughts and symptoms that arise. After a certain amount of time you could then re-score your anxiety levels to see if they've come down. You'll find - more often than not - that this happens.

Comparative scoring can also be helpful in situations that you may find difficult. Common examples include: being in a crowded place, travelling, social situations, health matters and even just being outside of the home. You can begin to take encouragement when you notice the overall or average levels of your anxiety decreasing.

Of course, not every occasion will provide a positive result because anxiety can vary in intensity. It is important not to take any notice or attach any importance to this if it ever occurs. Just keep going and your overall anxiety average will slowly decrease.

Lose the emotional crutches

In any stressful life it's common for someone to rely on little escapes and emotional crutches in order to get through the day. Common escapes include: smoking, drinking, recreational drugs, medication, computer games, over sleeping etc. I'm not here to discuss the pros and cons of doing such things, but I do feel these things can act as a stumbling block when they're completely relied upon as *emotional escapes*.

Common sayings such as *'I can't give up smoking because it would make everything worse'*, *'I'll always need this medication'*, *'I need a drink to ease the nerves'*, *'I'm just going to sleep it off'* are all small-scale examples of using an emotional crutch. To put it in basic terms, an emotional crutch is something we have irrationally concluded to be something we couldn't live without.

Personally, I don't see too many negatives in enjoying things such as drinking and smoking when in control and when they're a clear, conscious choice. However, when they're solely relied upon as a necessity for everyday life, then you'll find that they are used for reasons that go beyond enjoyment. An emotional crutch is essentially when a 'want' becomes a 'need' - much like an addiction.

A more profound example of an emotional crutch is when anxiety sufferers place so much importance on confining themselves to the walls of their homes. Home is suddenly this overtly safe place, where the walls suddenly become the mechanics of our mind and body's coping mechanisms. It's common to view the outside of the home as this dangerous and overwhelming place that our minds and bodies could not cope with. It's also very common to think that we can deal with our problems within our homes and essentially 'come out when we're ready'.

Emotional crutches are exclusive and subjective to the individual and I suggest that you take time out to distinguish between what you're enjoying and what you're actually relying on. On a personal note, I found that unhealthy habits such as smoking and binge drinking actually made my anxiety feel worse, with it only providing a short-term level of enjoyment or escape. Smoking actually over-stimulates the nervous system, making symptoms such as hypersensitivity and panic occur more frequently. Alcohol and the 'hang over' effect also cause similar symptoms and actually place us in states of vulnerability. Drinking alcohol drains our electrolyte levels which puts us at 'risk' of experiencing chest palpitations.

The best way to put yourself to the test with anxiety is to take yourself out of your comfort zone which, in most cases, is our homes. Lose the emotional crutches and see if you can go through a day without them. Of course, losing them all at once is a bit much to ask of yourself, so try and cut down on the bad habits a little bit of a time and see how you feel after a week.

If you're feeling agoraphobic, try and spend an hour going for a walk or seeing a friend. Why not cut down the cigarettes or other habitual drugs by half? Cutting down and eventually not having to rely on these emotional crutches did wonders for me when overcoming anxiety.

Keep fit, eat healthy

Any health professional will tell you that exercise and a healthy diet is paramount when establishing a good bill of health. This applies to dealing with anxiety too. It's well known that exercise and 'feel good' foods help with both physical and psychological ailments. With regards to anxiety, exercise and healthy foods are proven to ease the symptoms it produces. They can help ease symptoms such as heart palpitations, irritable bowel syndrome, poor blood circulation, tiredness and breathlessness to name a few.

Exercise helps to establish a good level of blood circulation, which helps to create efficient oxygen transportation and a good digestive cycle. It also helps the brain to release chemicals such as endorphins, which aid the body in experiencing the feeling of being happy and content. It also helps to provide an outlet for excessive adrenaline, which usually comes in abundance for the average anxiety sufferer.

Furthermore, it helps to add structure to our daily lives. Going for a run, cooking a healthy meal, going to the gym, doing household jobs or even going for a walk gives us a daily outlet for any negative feelings and helps to pull us out of negative thought patterns. Doing this, alongside eating healthier foods, has a huge, positive effect on mental health and I seriously recommend it. I believe it would help anyone just as much as it helped me.

The old saying of 'you are what you eat' rings true when it comes to choosing the right food. Eating nutritious, healthy foods which contain vitamins, calcium, protein and other essentials, not only aid us physically, but have been proven to help us mentally too. You should take time out to analyse and record which foods have a profound effect on your mood and how they affect you physically.

I decided to drastically cut down on my sugar intake, as well as wheat-based products, as I found that they negatively affected my mood and also made me feel bloated. They also made me feel lethargic and unmotivated - leaving me vulnerable for anxious thoughts to creep in. It's different for each individual and needs to be assessed using your own thoughts and feelings and the observations of those around you.

Here is a list of the common foods that seem to affect those with anxiety:

- **Wheat and food with high gluten content. i.e. Bread, dough,** - High wheat and gluten content in foods is known to trigger bloating, the symptoms of Irritable Bowel Syndrome, lethargy, stomach pains and chest tightness.
- **Sugar in high amounts. i.e. chocolate, sweets, cakes,** - High amounts of sugar intake can be linked to bloating, over-stimulates the nervous system, tiredness, lethargy and headaches.
- **Milk products. i.e. butter, cheese, cream,** - Dairy products can affect our digestion, cause I.B.S, bloating, trapped wind, lethargy, headaches and nausea.
- **Artificial additives. i.e. 'E numbers', food colourings, sweeteners,** - It takes the body longer to process artificial products. They can cause headaches, nausea, tiredness and can over-stimulate the nervous system.
- **Eggs.** - Eggs can drastically affect digestion speed causing indigestion and various other symptoms relating to I.B.S.
- **Spices.** - Spicy food can trigger digestion problems and I.B.S.

It's also widely advised that you cut down on red meat, as well as foods containing high fructose. Furthermore, you need to understand that meal sizes, particularly those consisting of large portions, can dramatically affect a person's mood. If we overeat, it causes our bodies to work harder to digest our food - affecting our energy levels.

All of the listed foods have been linked to triggering the symptoms of anxiety and they notably have the ability to lower our overall mood. Wheat and sugar particularly affected my energy levels and digestion, but it's all down to each individual and how their body reacts. For example, you may be affected by dairy products or eggs, but seem fine when eating other foods.

We know that anxiety can cause us to assume the worst-case scenario in a given situation. This is important to remember when seeing how our bodies react to foods. During my problems with anxiety, I assumed that I had something far-fetched such as coeliac disease, because I bloated after I ate bread and pizza. Perhaps you get stomach pain after drinking milk, so your anxious brain may assume that you're lactose intolerant.

Just remember that our anxious brains often *need* to find the answer and in doing so will jump to the easiest answer - the worst-case scenario. Anxiety has the power to cause I.B.S, bloating, lethargy, stomach pains etc. Just because you have the symptoms of a food intolerance doesn't mean you actually are permanently intolerant. It may just be anxiety. I recommend going to your general practitioner for a food intolerance test for assurance.

Foods which have been shown to provide a positive effect on anxious symptoms and overall mood are:

- **Fruit** - Bananas, apricots, apples, oranges, tomatoes, blueberries, avocados and various dried fruits such as sultanas, raisins and prunes to name a few.
- **Vegetables** - Broccoli, spinach, carrots, chickpeas, parsnips, beans, etc.
- **Nuts and Seeds** - Walnuts, almonds, pistachios, macadamias, Brazil nuts, pumpkin seeds, sunflower seeds, flax seeds, etc.
- **Grains** - oats, brown rice, corn, barley etc.
- **Oily fish** - Salmon, tuna, mackerel, sardines, herring etc.

These foods have all been linked to promoting increased mental health. If you're like me and can't resist eating animal meat, then try to stick to lean, white meats such as turkey and perhaps try to eat more fish. Experiment with your diet and record the benefits. This is particularly beneficial when our anxiety levels have improved and we want to continue our development.

Cut down on caffeine and alcohol

Caffeine can often be structured into our daily lives and relied upon as a means of providing 'instant' energy. It is a highly addictive stimulant that the body can crave when intake is stopped or lowered. Caffeine can be found in:

- Coffee
- Tea
- Soft Drinks
- Energy Drinks
- Painkillers

- Various medication

For anxiety sufferers, consuming caffeine can be very debilitating, as it can easily trigger anxious thoughts and symptoms. The aim, particularly with anxiety, is to slowly cut caffeine out of your diet until your anxiety becomes manageable or has subsided. I stress the importance of 'slowly', because those who have a high daily intake of caffeine are at risk of 'caffeine withdrawal'.

Caffeine is a stimulant that increases agitation and anxiety. It's also very acidic, which can lead to inflammation within the body. Caffeine is also a diuretic, which can lead to dehydration and worsen the other symptoms of anxiety.

I often drank coffee and tea as a quick fix to wake up in the morning, or to give myself an afternoon boost to help me focus at work. What I didn't realise was that it actually heightened the feeling of being anxious.

Not only does caffeine provide the feeling of increased energy levels, but it also stimulates our nervous system; this makes us prone to states of hypersensitivity and hyperawareness. We know that these are symptoms of anxiety that we'd much rather avoid. I strongly recommend aiming towards avoiding caffeine altogether and relying on healthier sources of energy such as fruit and high carbohydrate food.

Patience and discipline

You must be patient when trying to rid yourself of anxiety. If you use patience, perseverance and an alternate life focus, then the anxiety will eventually leave. Do not rush it, but at the same time do not let anxiety define who you are. In order to re-wire your brain to live a better life, you need to establish new habits. This takes time.

This book may have helped you to alleviate your initial fear of anxiety, but in order to truly eradicate it, you need to have a good sense of self-discipline and self-awareness. You need to be able to distinguish between what your true thoughts and beliefs are and those that are dictated by anxiety. When we are feeling 'fine', our outlook on life maybe positive and attributes such as our self-esteem, self-belief and motivation may not be questioned. However, when we're feeling anxious, we could think about these same attributes in a more negative light. It is up to you to distinguish which you truly believe in: the positive or the negative.

I think it's very important that you're not too hard on yourself when battling this condition. It's too easy to be our own worst critic during anxiety, but you need to realise that you're going through a lot of emotional trauma. There were many times where I thought I was doing well with regards to tackling my anxiety. I'd go weeks abiding by a routine that I knew was healthy for me and that I actually ended up engaging with.

But there were times where I did feel anxious. I did feel the onset of a panic attack. However, I acknowledged that it was simply anxiety trying to creep back in. It did get me down at times and on the odd occasion I felt like crumbling and accepting the label of being an anxious wreck. I persevered though and I insist that you do the same.

So, don't whirl up in a panic, or dwell on a depressive state if you feel your anxiety is troubling you. Always focus on the positives and constantly check on how far you've come. I fully believe that everyone with an anxiety disorder can overcome it. You must believe in that too.

The Do's and Do Not's when approaching anxiety

Do - Acknowledge that your symptoms are all connected to an anxiety problem. Group all of your worries under one umbrella and tackle them as one singular problem.

Do - Realise that when we feel panicky, lightheaded, wanting to escape or feel like something awful is going to happen, that this is primarily down to adrenaline and other bodily chemicals. The affect of your bodily chemicals have little connection to the outcomes of the outside world. Try and stick it out.

Do - Understand that anxiety comes with a lot of symptoms, which at times of high anxiety can seem completely separate from the issue at hand. However, if there is a concern then DO see your general practitioner for reassurance.

Do - Partake in what you would usually do or try something new. To begin re-wiring the brain, you must establish new positive thought paths and give the adrenal gland a rest. Do what you would usually do and keep your mind busy!

Do - Talk to people and be as open as you can about your anxiety. You'll find that those who care and love you will accept it in their own way and give you the space, time and patience you need to deal with the problem. This is great for relieving any pressures mounting in your social life.

Do - Look after your body by keeping it active and providing it with healthy foods.

Do Not - Accept that anxiety is simply who you are.

Do Not - Try to 'think your way out of it' in states of high anxiety. There is no 'miracle thought' that can cure all of your ailments.

Do Not - Assume the worst-case scenario. Anxiety and panic forces us to do this. Use positive rationalisation to realise that it's probably the anxiety, not your true beliefs.

Do Not - Run away from a situation. You'll only place more importance on the issue and make it become a more frightening prospect.

Do Not - Rely on emotional crutches, such as the walls of your own home, alcohol, drugs and even smoking.

Do Not - Do this alone. Share your thoughts, feelings, progress and experiences with others, regardless of what they think.

Do Not - Consume excessive amounts of caffeine and alcohol. Believe me on this one.

My story

WE HAVE REACHED THIS short and somewhat self-indulgent part of the book - my story with anxiety. This part of the book is an optional read, particularly if you're a closet misanthrope like me and cringe at any sign of someone appearing to bask in their own self-involvement. I do feel telling my story is helpful though, as it provides you with an idea about what I went through with my battle with anxiety. It may also provide you with hope as I've been there; I've done it.

My anxiety first started when I left university and was left heavily in debt. I had no job and I was trying to maintain a failing long-distance relationship. I'd also made the decision to quit a pretty destructive cannabis habit (cannabis does not help in the long run).

I felt a bit lost. I didn't know what to do and felt out of my comfort zone. I was worrying about what the future held for me. I was worrying about money, my relationship, where I would live, my old friendships being re-kindled and if I could adapt to my new environment.

It was my first year out of university. I was living with my mum and younger brother and trying my best to establish myself in the world. I suffered with what can be labeled as *generalised anxiety* and often spent my days dwelling on why I felt so edgy, so different.

I realised that dwelling on my problems wasn't healthy, so I put all of my effort into getting a job, so I could have financial security and an ability to see my partner and my friends more often. It also kept my mind busy.

After a short while, I managed to get a job as a support worker for disabled adults, which I found very rewarding, although there were periods of time in the working day that allowed me to dwell on my worries.

After a year, with my worries still the same, I decided that I needed a change. I had almost saved enough money to move into my own place and thought it would help with my generalised anxiety. I loved living with my family, particularly my younger brother, as he was at that fun age of 14 where he helped me to re-live some of my past times, but the mental associations I held about living at home were not helping my anxiety.

I managed to get a better job in a career I always wanted to be involved in. I felt hope. My relationships improved, my anxiety lessened, my social life flourished and I had the opportunity and financial means to move out and start an independent life.

A month before I was due to start my new job, my younger brother was diagnosed with an extremely rare form of cancer. The odds were simply astronomical. My family were in shock and the trauma hit us all hard. I had to stay home and look after my brother and my mum. The trauma of his diagnosis hit me very, very hard. As for the anxiety, well, I'm sure you can imagine. For two years I stayed in my family home and cared for my mum and brother.

Now I will explain, strictly from an anxiety point of view, what the effects of anxiety did to me during this difficult time. I realise I run the risk of sounding somewhat selfish, given that I wasn't the one with the serious illness, but this book is ultimately about anxiety and I will focus strictly on that.

Immediately after my brother's diagnosis and in my alone time, I began to think and obsess about the concept of death. My main environments were now my home and a children's oncology ward. I was so adamant that I was going to help my brother that I made my whole life about cancer. I wanted to know everything in order to 'save' my brother. Please bear in mind that I already struggled with generalised anxiety.

I couldn't sleep, my brain was in overdrive and all my thoughts about the trauma where on a constant loop. I meticulously analysed and emotionally smothered my brother. I was acting out of panic. Subsequently my relationship with my partner and certain friends broke down. I began to feel more and more isolated, without even acknowledging it, because my focus was so narrow.

After a discussion with my mum, I decided to proceed to undertake the new job I was due to start, as a means of keeping my mind focused and occupied on other things. This helped my panic-inducing thought patterns immeasurably, but what I failed to do was take some time out to look after myself. My life ultimately ended up being a hectic routine of working, helping my family and dwelling on illness, abandonment and replaying the trauma over and over again in my head. I kept this up for a few months, up until my body had simply had enough.

The breakdown happened.

I was at work one day making myself a hot drink, when all of a sudden I experienced a sudden wave of what can only be described as a complete detachment from my surroundings. My peripheral vision shut down, my breathing altered, my reality appeared distorted and everything seemed more lucid than real. *'What on earth is happening to me?'* I thought.

I began to panic.

It was the start of the mother of all panic attacks.

I was taken home.

For the next five days I locked myself in my room - unable to eat and sleep, experiencing the same level of panic that I had left work with. My mind was in overdrive and I just spent every minute panicking about why I felt the way I did. I couldn't sleep due to excessive worry and often spent my time trying to work out what I was going through. I would not leave the house, speak to anybody or even attempt to do anything that was required in my daily life.

Out of desperation I began to trawl the internet. I attempted to read articles and researched my symptoms everywhere I could find them. Each and every search ended up feeding me a worst-case scenario. After two days of feeling perpetually worse, I began to ponder on the possibility that I was going insane - that some incurable, psychological condition was causing my problems and that I was potentially brain damaged. What made it worse was that when I was searching the internet, I had read about many others who were going through the same thing. Some of these people, who had been living with similar symptoms, had been crippled by fear for years.

This added further stress to my already exhausted body. I was trying to fend off the possibility that I was mentally ill, as well as feeling a deep level of guilt about not being able to care for my brother and my mum. Thoughts just kept playing on loop in my brain. I felt completely immobilised. Then to make things worse, the anxiety started to affect me physically.

I started to get headaches, chest pains, breathing difficulties, heart palpitations, dizziness and this overwhelming sense of being far away from my surroundings. My stomach and ribs began to hurt, I could not keep still and I found focusing on anything to be near impossible. This carried on for weeks. I began to consider giving up. I considered running away (even though I didn't want to leave the house). I considered accepting that I was going insane. I considered suicide and all sorts of thoughts revolving around 'escaping'.

One night, when I was particularly panicky and hadn't slept or eaten for three days, I decided to walk to an old friend's house down the road. My friend was surprised when I turned up but allowed me to come in and talk about what I was going through. She listened attentively and after explaining about my predicament, she said something so subtle yet so profound it actually helped to kick start my recovery. *"Well it's no wonder you're having all of this anxiety."* she said.

Of all the racing thoughts and scenario conjurations my mind had processed, not one of them stopped to contemplate that it was just anxiety. Exhausted, I went home and once again tried to piece together a mental puzzle, but I used anxiety as the missing piece. It was a theory that had no flaw. That night I had the best sleep I'd had in a long while.

Don't be under any illusion that all my problems with anxiety suddenly ceased to exist just because I realised that it was 'just anxiety'. What it did do for me was provide me with a platform and a direct and harmless excuse to point all of my problems towards. My life was extremely stressful and I always reminded myself about what my friend said –'*no wonder I'm having all of this anxiety'*. Every time I felt panicky, experienced a physical symptom or noticed that my mind wondered off down a negative thought route, I just blamed it on anxiety.

This was the catalyst for overcoming my excessive anxiety. I did my research, put into practice the strategies and knowhow that you have found in this book and began to just get on with life. I once again became a big help to my family and helped my brother to tackle his illness. I saw friends, my attendance at work significantly improved and I even managed to set some leisure time for myself.

During his illness, I once asked my brother why he never seemed to panic about the severity of the situation. I couldn't understand why I seemed to reach this point of breakdown, whilst he always seemed to keep his cool and get on with things. The truth be told - the boy didn't know. To me he was this immortal figure of endless bravery, with such bravery seemingly a part of him.

After much thought, I realised this belief didn't serve him any justice. The boy actually made the conscious choice to be brave and kept himself mentally healthy through his own actions. This truly inspired me to replicate the same approach. I wanted to be brave and allow my *actions* to dictate my mentality.

I miss him to this day.

There's always hope for this condition. I now live a life almost free from it. I wish you all the best and please feel free to contact me to let me know your story.

PART 4

Emergency Panic Attack Help Page

IF YOU CURRENTLY FEEL like you're very anxious, or perhaps are panicking at this very moment, then read on and refer to these pages if panic ever strikes again.

OK, so you're panicking...

Let me guess:

Racing thoughts?

Feelings of terror, doom and even fear of death? Feel like you're going insane?

I know it feels horrible. I've had many panic attacks myself.

You need to realise that **nothing bad is going to happen** to you.

Absolutely nothing.

Your thoughts at this moment in time are merely a projection of your fears.

...this is not the reality of the situation.

You will calm down eventually.

You may not know this but there's a tonne of **adrenaline** and **cortisol** flowing through your veins at this very moment.

They're **harmless bodily chemicals.** You're in no danger.

You have entered **'fight or flight'** mode. You are in no danger.

None at all.

Soon the adrenaline will run out. I know this because the adrenal gland exhausts itself.

Your body can't maintain this panic.

It's biologically impossible.

I'm going to assume that you feel like this panic has come out of nowhere and that it feels out of your control.

You are fine.

This is normal.

Do not run away.

It is just the adrenaline. You are in 'fight or flight' mode.

Do you feel very different?

Does everything around you feel different?

They should do, because this is normal at a time like this.

It's just the adrenaline.

Is your mind racing?

A thousand thoughts a second?

Fearing the worst of your predicament?

This is also normal at a time like this.

It's just the adrenaline.

I bet this has happened before, perhaps many a time.

I bet this panic feels just as overwhelming as the other occasions that you've panicked, despite the previous experiences that you've had.

Wherever you are and whatever you're doing, you need to realise that nothing 'bad' is going to happen.

Believe me on this one.

I know how hard it is to 'think straight' when dealing with panic.

All you need to know is that your body has released a lot of harmless adrenaline into your system. Also, your **nervous system** is on **high alert**.

You have entered 'fight or flight' mode.

It's just the adrenaline.

This is normal.

This 'fight or flight' mode causes all sorts of **changes in the mind and body**.

It distorts our reality, makes our **heart beat fast,** makes us **shake, sweat** and **shiver**.

Believe me when I say that adrenaline can cause so many temporary, harmless changes within the body.

It does not matter if you chose to enter fight or flight mode or not. It is happening, and it will pass quickly if you **acknowledge** what is going on within your body.

Steady your breathing, let the adrenaline pass and let the **nervous system settle**.

This feeling will pass soon.

Look forward to the fact that when the adrenal gland exhausts itself, it brings a feeling of light euphoria to the mind and body.

Look forward to this - it is a **truly amazing feeling**.

Keep doing what you were supposed to be doing, whether you're at home, at work, travelling or even on holiday.

The feeling will eventually pass.

Do not show this feeling the attention that it does not deserve. Continue with your day and if the feeling ever strikes again, it will not be as intense as this time - I guarantee.

Keep active and **focus on something positive**. This is hard, but even thinking about something positive **diverts the negative thoughts** your mind is homing in on.

Everything will be fine. Nothing bad is going to happen.

Nothing bad *can* happen.

You can do it.

It's just the adrenaline.

By the same author...

Anxiety: Practical about Panic

I SINCERELY HOPE THAT you have enjoyed this book and hopefully taken something positive from it. If you are interested in any further reading, then please feel free to read my second book, *Anxiety: Practical about Panic*, which was written a few years after this. The second book contains added information that has been derived and collated from my work at The Panic Room, as well as invaluable knowledge obtained from Master's level study in Counselling Psychology. You can find Practical about Panic online, or it can be found in several well-known book stores.

Many thanks for reading.

Made in the USA
Monee, IL
16 October 2022

16009947R00090

EAT VEGAN
with Me

Creating Community through
Conversation and Compassionate Cuisine

Mary Lawrence

2017

Danvers

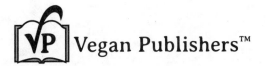 Vegan Publishers™

To everyone who makes a difference by shining their light on the truth, standing up for those who are exploited and oppressed, and refusing to give in or give up, with all of my heart I thank you. You are brave heroes.

Vegan Publishers
Danvers, Massachusetts
www.veganpublishers.com

© 2017 by Mary Lawrence

All rights reserved. No part of this book may be reproduced or transmitted in any form or by any means, electronic or mechanical, without written permission.

Photography by Annika Lundqvist Photography

Cover and text design by Nicola May Design

All products mentioned in this book are trademarks of their respective companies. No claims of endorsement are made by including these products.

♻ Printed in the United States of America on 100% recycled paper

First edition, paperback

ISBN: 978-1-940184-44-9

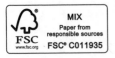

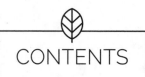

CONTENTS

Acknowledgements IX

Dedication XI

Introduction XIII

How to Use This Book XVII

PART 1

Chapter 1 Coming Out as Vegan 3

Chapter 2 A Seat at the (Vegan) Table 11

Chapter 3 Overcoming Obstacles 21

Chapter 4 Socializing 33

Chapter 5 Becoming a Vegan Gardener 45

Chapter 6 Self-care for the Vegan Activist 55

Chapter 7 Dress for Success 67

Chapter 8 The Vegan Kitchen 81

PART 2

Chapter 9 Recipes 101

Breakfast 105

Lunch 125

Dinner 161

Desserts 223

Cooking Conversions 251

Recipe Index 255

Appendix – Resources 259

About the Author 263

Acknowledgements

First and foremost, I am incredibly grateful for the love and support of my parents, Joe and Fran Lawrence, who have been with me on this 20-year vegan journey. I feel so fortunate that I get to share my experiences with them, and that every day our relationship grows stronger and richer. I'm also thrilled that on my brother's 50th birthday, he announced that he hadn't eaten meat in 3 weeks! Thank you, Joey, for moving in the vegan direction, and for taking care of yourself.

Thank you to Dr. Casey Taft of Vegan Publishers who came to my presentation, "Cooking Vegan for Non-vegan Family and Friends," and thought it would make a good topic for a cookbook. Everywhere I go, people tell me this is their greatest challenge when becoming vegan, and I hope that reading this book will help make it a little easier. Thank you also to my fabulous recipe testers and focus group participants: Susan Armknecht, Carol Belau, Christine Cioffi, Jessica Greenebaum, Karen James, Wes Kasprow, Patty Mondo, Judy Panciera, Cora Perrone, Devin Pray, Anita Rebarchak, Amy Grammatica Rios, Lorena Salas, Jessica Sokol, Patricia Canning Stevens, Garrett Taylor, and Erika Ueberbacher. Your feedback helped make these recipes ROCK!

I also want to thank everyone who is part of the growing vegan community, both here in Connecticut and all over the world. I'm honored to meet so many compassionate and dedicated people in my travels as well as online who are working together to create the world we want to live in. You inspire me every day.

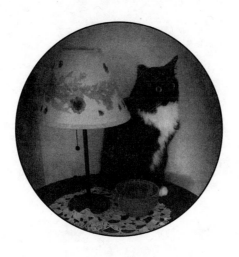

Dedication

To my sweet ray of sunshine, my sanctuary, my angel kitty who blessed me with four-and-a-half years of pure love and joy, I dedicate this book to you. Gremlin (aka, Gerrrrbs Grems Prince Poppy Seed Purr Machine), from the day Zinny and I found you on the side of the road as a tiny kitten barely clinging to life, you filled my heart with immense joy, and you made me feel like the luckiest person in the world. So many chapters of this book were written during the dark days of winter, huddled under our favorite blankie, with you snuggled by my side. Your purrs were the best therapy. You're the first kitty I ever shared my life with, and I'm so incredibly grateful for every moment we had together and for everything you taught me.

Hug and kiss your precious ones for us, and savor every moment with those you love.

Introduction

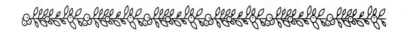

There are two things nearly every vegan I know has in common: 1) they never thought they could ever be vegan and 2) their only regret is that they didn't become vegan sooner. Sound familiar? Ever since we were little children, we connected almost instinctively with our love of animals, and most of us were also taught by our parents not to harm them. You'd think naturally that would make us all vegan, right? The reality we know, however, is far from the case. Just as we pick up the language of our culture, we also assimilate what is "appropriate" and "normal" behavior through our daily routine, a routine that is centered around three meals a day. Years of socialization inevitably lead us to adopt similar habits to those around us as we establish our place in our families, circle of friends, workplace, and eventually the world, and those habits typically include eating meat and animal products. We drop our instinctive love of animals in favor of a more acceptable and convenient disassociation in order to fit in. Being perceived as "different" is a label we're conditioned to avoid, so we follow along with prescribed traditions instead and quiet our questioning minds.

Despite our social conditioning, most of us retain that sense of wonder with the natural world and connection to animals into adulthood. We love our dogs, cats, and other companion animals and consider them family members. Some of us even rescue homeless animals and take in fosters so that they can be rehabilitated and find loving forever homes. This altruism is an expression of who we are as caring, compassionate people, not for our own benefit, but for the selfless act of helping another who is in need.

As vegans, we rebel against social conditioning and reconnect with our true compassionate nature, committing ourselves to live in alignment with the values we were taught as children. We follow The Golden Rule, "do unto others as you would have them do unto you," because we believe it to be fair and just. We adopt a lifestyle that resonates with our belief that, in the words of The Vegan Society founder Donald Watson, "seeks to exclude—as far as is possible and practicable—all forms of exploitation of, and cruelty to, animals for food, clothing, or any other purpose, and by extension, promotes the development and use of animal-free alternatives for the benefit of humans, animals, and the environment." This noble lifestyle is perceived as admirable by some, and unattainable by many. But we know it is simply a matter of living with authenticity and integrity.

Although there is philosophical consensus that compassion is a desirable trait and veganism is worth aspiring to, in practice we often find ourselves alone. Many of us are the "lone vegan" in our families and circle of friends. We often feel isolated, alone, frustrated, and even betrayed. Some of us choose to keep our veganism hidden from even our closest relationships for fear of being ostracized or ridiculed. We master various coping mechanisms for social situations where other people don't even give a second of thought. We call it a "diet" or an "allergy" to imply our food choice is something we have no control over because that let's us off the hook to scrutiny. We try not to inconvenience anyone and apologize for our special meal requests. We use the term "plant-based" so that others won't feel threatened or judged. We learn to "make do," "get by," and "make excuses" rather than unintentionally impose our beliefs on others. We avoid uttering "the v word" because it's easier to just say, "no thank you, I'm not hungry." All of this is great for getting along with people, minimizing conflict, and maintaining our relationships, but we are not being true to ourselves, and our lack of authenticity invariably creates an internalized moral dilemma.

In polite society we are expected to "put up and shut up," to tolerate actions by others that we find repugnant. These daily lessons in social etiquette may win us popularity contests if we obey the rules, but they do nothing to change the status quo of animal exploitation. Do we silence ourselves for the sake of acquiescing to our family and friends, or do we speak up and risk social stigma? It's time we turn the tables.

Eat Vegan with Me brings vegan ethics to the dinner table and demonstrates how to navigate tricky social situations while staying true to your values. There is no space for excuses, apologies, or complicity when we're trying to change the world! As vegan activists, we must be proactive in demonstrating appropriate behavior in our daily interactions. We can no longer choose silence if we want to end the unnecessary violence and needless exploitation of animals in our society. We must stop apologizing for the truth, tolerating injustice, and compromising our values in order to create the world we want to live in. This is not simply a cookbook, but rather a recipe for vegans who want to transform the dinner table and effect positive social change in the world.

When we come together in unity with compassion for ourselves and all beings, we can heal the planet. We can empower ourselves and each other to create a global vegan community that represents a new social norm based on compassion and justice, not exploitation and violence. As we grapple with these issues and develop confidence in the kitchen, never again will we feel the need to apologize for making compassion the main course.

How to Use This Book

First of all, let me thank you for picking up this book. I'm hoping it's because you've shared similar experiences as I have had trying to convince family and friends to become vegan. Maybe you've felt frustrated defending your veganism to everyone. Or despite being adept at fielding every possible question about nutrition, animals, and the environment, you still feel ineffective at motivating others to change. Whatever the reason, your journey has led you to continue to search for answers here.

On the surface this is a cookbook, but think of it as much more. Sure, there are some delicious recipes you'll enjoy making and sharing. Beyond that, consider each chapter in this book a step-by-step guide for how to take charge of interactions with non-vegan family and friends and become a powerful force for change. You are a positive voice for animals within your own social circles. That is a position to be proud of. Always know that you are making a difference in the world simply by being a vegan role model in everything that you do. But if you'd like to have more of an impact, please read on.

In this book you will learn how to transform social situations by engaging in honest, direct communication, staying poised and focused on your message, being mindful of each person's needs, visualizing desired outcomes, and becoming a confident and competent chef, to ultimately enable your loved ones to make the vegan transition. You will identify your greatest challenges, set goals and action steps for overcoming obstacles, and create positive affirmations to focus your intentions on a daily basis. As you work on these techniques, you will discover your relationships changing and growing in ways you never before imagined possible.

Over the past 13 years I have used my experience as a college educator and public speaker, passion as an animal activist, and expertise as executive chef of my vegan personal chef service, Well on Wheels, to help hundreds of people lead healthy, happy lives or recover from a wide variety of health problems by transitioning to a vegan lifestyle. I have worked with everyone from children to senior citizens, urban and rural populations, economically disadvantaged and physically challenged, teaching them that food can be healthy, affordable, and delicious without harming animals. What they have learned and what you will learn, too, are strategies that enable behavior change. Nearly 99% of the population say they love animals, but getting them to put their beliefs into action by not harming them through their food choices is a skill that you will develop by following the strategies detailed in this book.

If you've ever felt concerned that others don't share your values and the world will never be vegan, let me reassure you that there is hope. I've seen people change, and the reverberation of these transformations has so much potential for massive culture shift. As you put these practices into action, you will gain self-confidence and determination to turn your empathy into activism for the animals by guiding your loved ones not just to a better life for themselves, but to a better world for all beings.

Part 1

Conversations

Chapter 1

Coming Out as Vegan

Any major change begins with the first step. For many of us, the decision to become vegan was a long, thought-out process that required extensive self-examination, months of research, scrutinizing every single ingredient label, trial and error in the kitchen, and endless deliberation over what our friends and families would think. If we were lucky, we had someone to go through it with us, or at least a supportive confidant who encouraged us to persevere. The reality, however, is that many of us make the transition alone. We happen into it without advanced preparation, not expecting the repercussions that often ensue. Although we are 100% committed to the moral and ethical reasons behind our decision, we feel unsure of our ability to defend it when interrogated by those who expect us to suddenly become experts in nutrition, human biology, environmental sustainability, and animal behavior.

The process of adapting to or adopting new cultural patterns (e.g., beliefs, practices, traits, and habits) of a dominant group is known as "acculturation."[1] Traditionally, this is a process whereby non-native immigrants assimilate into a dominant culture, but the experience of adopting a vegan lifestyle can share similar hurdles, such as education, access to and availability of ingredients, learning new cooking methods, time to adjust, and affordability. Acculturation occurs in two stages. At the micro (individual) level are the psychological changes in attitudes, beliefs, and behaviors of the individual in transition. At the macro (group) level, physical, political, economic, and cultural changes occur within the vegan's personal sphere. We will explore these aspects of acculturation in this chapter.

Making the Decision to Go Vegan

We all have an experience that led us to that vegan fork in the road. For me, it was a health crisis that started me on this path. It was 1997, a time when being vegan wasn't very popular, and those who had heard the word identified it as a diet. This was an easy association for me because I had done a complete overhaul of my diet due to health reasons. I was sick all the time with allergies, asthma, a chronic cough, migraines, unexplained rashes, debilitating fatigue, and numerous digestive issues. Traditional doctors told me I was allergic to pet dander and gave me two instructions: get rid of my dog and take medication for the rest of my life. Because I was skeptical of anyone who would suggest I part with a family member and I didn't want to be a slave to the pharmaceutical industry, I decided to seek other treatment options. This began my journey learning about alternative medicine, nutrition, and how food can affect one's health. My life and my health completely turned around as a result. That was acceptable to my friends and family who

---

1. Satiaabouta, J., et al. *"Dietary acculturation: Applications to nutrition research and dietetics."* Journal of the American Dietetic Association, vol. 102, no. 8, 2002, pp. 1105–1118.

wanted the best for me, believing that this diet was only temporary until I recovered.

I also started eating more mindfully, which made me keenly aware of where my food came from, including the food I once ate. After a visit to Farm Sanctuary in 2002, I met the lucky few who were saved from lives of suffering and eventual slaughter, and I became committed to ethical vegan activism as a result. My entire belief system was changing. Once my eyes were opened, I wanted to share what I learned with the world. Many of us who go vegan for ethical reasons take it upon ourselves to become activists and educate others. It became my personal mission to share what I knew with as many people as possible, and I decided at that moment to dedicate my life to speaking out about the cruelties of the animal agriculture industry and to demonstrate how a vegan lifestyle is the ethical solution to ending unnecessary violence.

That is the approach I took with everyone I knew. I naively believed that surely, if they heard what I had to say and read the literature I shared, they would instantly see the light and want to go vegan as well. My family and friends are all kind, caring people. They're well-educated, intelligent, and honest. They were raised the same way I was, to be kind to animals. I expected our next dinner together to include a frank discussion about animal suffering and our exploitative food system while foregoing meatballs in favor of chowing down some vegan lasagna. Alas, that wasn't the case.

In reality, what I faced was a brick wall. In some instances there was acknowledgement followed by resignation: "Yes, it's horrible, but it's too big of a problem for us to fix." In others there was resentment and hostility: "You're going to ruin dinner for us!" These are reactions that many of us face when we announce our decision to be vegan. We may also open up deep psychological wounds, discover bullies lurking in our circles, have our efforts sabotaged, or be excommunicated from our closest relationships.

All of these are possibilities when we confront social norms, but they are not to be taken personally. Ethical veganism invites a close examination of our daily habits that many are unwilling to undertake, particularly when it's thrust upon them. Because of this, it's important that we recognize certain possible reactions and be prepared to manage them *before* they happen.

Conversations with Family and Friends

Being open and honest with our family and friends is crucial in the moment we first begin discussing our intentions to become vegan. It is a serious matter that involves much introspection, and it is important that we indicate to our loved ones the significance of this decision. Even if you're a long-time vegan still struggling with these issues, it's possible to reassert your intentions in a new light. Setting ground rules that will ensure your ability to succeed is crucial, and what works best will depend on one's individual comfort level. These might include:

> » What products are allowed in the home, kitchen, bath, and beyond
> » Grocery shopping and stocking the vegan pantry
> » Dining out with non-vegans
> » Special occasions and holiday get-togethers
> » Conversations about food, animals, the environment, and social justice issues
> » Respectful behaviors that demonstrate support

Each of these will be discussed further in Chapter 2 when we put our behaviors into practice. For now, it is important to begin with a basic list of guidelines that can help navigate interpersonal dynamics and minimize conflict. It's also important in these conversations to recognize the feelings of others. Whether they're supportive or defensive, pleased or pissed off, know that you are not to blame for their reactions. Change is difficult for all of us, and even indirectly there will be adjustments in everyone's lives. Adding to one's daily stresses can feel overwhelming. Be sure to recognize the feelings of others and acknowledge their validity with reassuring words while also expressing your needs. Try using variations on the following statements to empathize with these concerns:

> *"I understand that this may be difficult for you to accept."*
>
> *"Yes, this is a big change that affects all of us, and I appreciate your support and understanding."*
>
> *"It may seem like a tremendous hurdle right now, but we can make this work."*
>
> *"It's important to me that we're able to maintain our relationship."*

One of the reasons why it's so hard to win over family members to veganism is because in order to do so we have to break rank. This causes a disruption to family dynamics that many people can't understand and have a difficult time adjusting to. The most they can do is be politely accommodating out of a sense of loyalty to the family structure, but to do anything more—to join in that disruption by becoming an ally— may pose too great a risk to them of tearing apart the fabric holding the family together. They don't want to be an accomplice to such a social crime. Accept that some tension is inevitable no matter how positive you may be in communicating your intentions. Trust that this will eventually subside and interactions will become less fraught with anxiety over time.

Speaking Your Truth

One of the most difficult challenges to being vegan is not only standing up for animals, but standing up for ourselves. In our society we are taught to make compromises for the greater good, particularly if we're women. We condition ourselves to be people pleasers so that others will like us. We just want to get along after all! Doing something contrary to social norms, like becoming vegan, can put us in a position where we feel the need to explain ourselves and justify our actions so that others won't be offended. This is a social response known as "saving face," where we attempt to alleviate others' discomfort by redirecting blame to ourselves so that we can maintain their respect. When you sense this happening, always remind yourself that being vegan is about compassion for all living beings and aligning one's behaviors with those beliefs. That is nothing to apologize for. Further, a certain amount of discomfort is necessary in order to be a catalyst for change. Recognize others' concerns, but always stay true to yourself.

Keep in mind the words of Walt Whitman, "I and mine do not convince by arguments, similes, rhymes. We convince by our presence." Being honest, open, and direct in a society that so often camouflages painful truths with palatable lies can be a difficult skill to learn at first, but it eventually becomes easier. Once you begin unraveling layers of ambiguity and deception, exposing the reality in which we live becomes inevitable. As a vegan, it is distressing to become aware of the hatred, violence, and suffering in the world and to be exposed to the seemingly unfathomable depths of depravity, but as enlightened citizens of this planet it is our moral obligation to not only be informed, but act upon that knowledge. Most of us were once meat eaters, whether willful or ignorant, or willfully ignorant. Some may have even believed the humane myth because we were desensitized to, or disconnected from, the inherent violence in the industry. I think back to who I was before I became aware of this cruelty and the kind of person I wish I had met that would influence me to go vegan, and I try to be that person today. For me, those who gave me honest, direct information shared with sensitivity and understanding, free of judgment and condemnation, made me stop in my tracks and want to change. By standing strong with our convictions, we disempower the saboteurs and empower ourselves to create the world we want to live in. Let us always remember to speak up even when our voice is shaking, and never apologize for promoting kindness and nonviolence. When you speak the truth, you discover you're not alone.

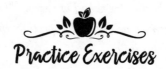

Practice Exercises

In this chapter we explored the practice of aligning actions with beliefs, breaking the news of becoming vegan to family and friends, setting ground rules for our interactions, and being assertive in conversations. Use the following exercises to describe where you are in that process and create a plan for overcoming obstacles you currently face.

CHALLENGES

Describe your life as a vegan right now, including the challenges you face. (*e.g., unsupportive parents, hostile family members, significant other who is not vegan, anxiety in social situations, etc.*)

SETTING GOALS

Determine 3 to 5 changes you would like to happen that would improve your interpersonal relationships. (*e.g., acceptance of your being vegan, ease of communication with difficult people, former non-vegans demonstrate empathy by becoming vegan, develop confidence as a vegan activist, etc.*)

ACTION STEPS
What can you do to make these goals a reality? *(e.g., set up meeting to discuss ground rules, write a letter explaining how you feel, cook a delicious vegan meal for non-vegans, practice positive self-care to minimize stress, etc.)*

POSITIVE AFFIRMATIONS
Envision your life in the future after these goals are achieved and make "present tense" statements describing it. *(e.g., "My parents are supportive of my veganism. They are happy I'm a compassionate person." "Conversations with non-vegans are easy. I enjoy letting them know why I'm vegan." "I'm so happy my best friend decided to become vegan. I appreciate that she understands how important this is.")*

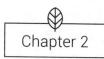

Chapter 2

A Seat at the (Vegan) Table

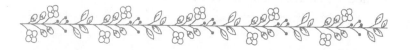

Once you've come out as vegan, there will inevitably be difficult conversations with family and friends that ensue. Have no fear! It is rare that everyone is instantly accepting, although we are grateful when they are. Stating what is acceptable behavior not only makes it clear to others what you will and won't tolerate, but it establishes your position of power at the table. Wait. What? A vegan with power?! It took me years to learn this and yes, in retrospect, I wish I had realized much sooner that I could empower myself in social situations by simply asserting myself. I was too preoccupied worrying about reactions like "who does she think she is?!" and being labeled the "angry vegan" or "pushy" to recognize that these are common misperceptions when anyone steps outside of social norms. At their worst, these responses silence us from speaking the truth and maintain the status quo. So speak up! Tell them what you want! Remember, you have a choice to either take what you get or get what you take. It's always prefer-able to take charge of the situation rather than wait for someone to tell you there's nothing vegan on the menu.

Black feminist civil rights activist Audre Lorde conveyed the need to speak out and take action in order to create social change in her essay, "The Transformation of Silence into Language and Action."[1] It's important not just for imploring justice, but for self-actualization. She wrote, "the transformation of silence into language and action is an act of self-revelation and that always seems fraught with danger. But my daughter, when I told her of our topic and my difficulty with it, said, 'tell them about how you're never really a whole person if you remain silent, because there's always that one little piece inside of you that wants to be spoken out, and if you keep ignoring it, it gets madder and madder and hotter and hotter, and if you don't speak it out one day it will just up and punch you in the mouth.'"

Speaking Your Truth

While we can't account for every conversation that may arise, we can prepare in advance for many by asking ourselves a series of questions that will help us be effective communicators. What do I need to stay true to my values? What will make me the most comfortable in this particular situation? What are the potential repercussions of this interaction? Our needs vary from one individual to the next and often depend on the context of a situation, but minimally we should always strive to establish dialogue that is both honest and kind. This can require a great deal of soul-searching when confronted by someone who is antagonistic. In some cases, self-preservation may be the best option. We all have different emotional thresholds when it comes to disagreements, where some are easily flooded with emotion from any type of conflict, while others can get into screaming matches

---

1. Lorde, Audre, and Cheryl Clarke. *Sister outsider: essays and speeches.* Berkeley: Crossing Press, 2007.

without feeling the least bit perturbed. One's comfort level might depend on calling for a "time out" period to step away from the conversation to be continued at a later, agreed upon time. Another ground rule could be an agreement to ban raised voices, name calling, accusations, and other dismissive behaviors. The following are some options to consider discussing and agreeing upon in advance with loved ones:

> **In the Home**: maintaining a vegan kitchen; stocking the pantry and refrigerator with only vegan products; cooking vegan at home; eliminating leather, wool, and other products made from animals; donating non-perishable food items and clothing made with animal products.

> **Shopping:** purchasing only cruelty-free health and beauty products; buying only vegan food items from the grocery store; buying produce from farmers markets and Community Supported Agriculture (CSA); shopping on-line vegan retailers; buying clothing and other household items made without wool, silk, or leather.

> **Dining Out:** frequenting only vegetarian restaurants; ordering only vegan menu items at non-vegan restaurants and requesting non-vegans not order animal products; requesting restaurants and food service establishments add vegan items to their menus; not dining where the bodies of animals are being served.

> **Special Occasions**: bringing vegan food to family get-togethers; eating vegan before the event; attending the event but abstaining from eating where

animals' bodies are served; hosting a vegan dinner party for special occasions.

Assertive Communication Techniques

Whatever the situation may be, it's always important to speak honestly and directly, and without judgment or sarcasm. Certainly there are times when your patience is tested and it's easy to reflexively respond with a caustic remark, but this will only do damage to not only your relationship but also your credibility. Remember, there is no need to be defensive when you are speaking the truth. Sometimes the most disarming response we can give to someone who is antagonistic is to ask, "Does my being vegan make you uncomfortable?" This redirects attention to the other person so that you are not in a position to be defensive. It's not your responsibility to address insults or jokes made at your expense, nor fuel a debate that is only intended to avoid self-examination. If a conversation threatens to become emotionally heated, take a few seconds to step back, take a deep breath, collect your thoughts, and mentally repeat one of your positive affirmations before proceeding. *"Conversations with non-vegans are easy. I am a positive role model."*

It is helpful to practice non-verbal behaviors that demonstrate confidence and reinforce your message. For example:

- » Make soft eye contact to show you care.
- » Nod your head with the person you are speaking with to show understanding, not necessarily agreement.
- » Maintain an upright yet relaxed body posture.
- » Lean toward the person you are speaking with.
- » Whenever appropriate, smile.

Breaking the Silence While Breaking Bread

Even at the dinner table, it's possible to discuss veganism with non-vegans, and we shouldn't shy away from it. In fact, respectful, informative conversations about food at the dinner table may be one of the few opportunities to raise the ethical aspects of veganism as it relates to the exploitation of animals, the environment, farm and slaughterhouse workers, and other social justice issues. This practice used to be taboo, much like talking about politics or religion, because of its sensitive nature. However, once the ground rules are established and respected, it's only logical that food will be discussed when dining together. Why should we be silent about something that matters so much to us? As vegan Democratic Senator from New Jersey Corey Booker says, "In the cause of justice: never stay silent just so that others can remain comfortable."

Always remember to be respectful in tone, respond to sincere questions with honesty and kindness, and share your story. The most compelling response to any inquiry is to provide your personal experience. For one, it can't be disputed. But more importantly, allowing yourself to be vulnerable in this way establishes an emotional bond with the questioner. We live in a society where people tend to be much more comfortable being physically naked than emotionally naked, and many people hide behind various masks in order to feel safe. Your authenticity can have a powerful impact in that it demonstrates courage to break free of these facades and be true to yourself. Encourage that in others. In many cases, your greatest detractors may be those who are struggling to break free from playing roles that don't fit them.

Managing Emotions and Maintaining Balance

By expressing your wants and needs, you can overcome many emotional triggers. "I need you to listen for a minute" or "I want to talk about something important to me" are assertive statements that can be used to begin a conversation about veganism, or focus one that has gotten off track. When these wishes are respected, a positive tone is set from the start and the discussion can proceed with equanimity. However, there are times when we're met with sarcasm or even hostility and mocking responses such as "Oh no, what now?!" accompanied by eye rolls and closed ears. This is when it's important to exercise true empathy by acknowledging the other person's unwillingness to engage in a difficult conversation, but nonetheless continuing to assert its necessity. For example:

> *Vegan:* "Can we discuss how we'll cook vegan in our kitchen? This is really important to me."
>
> *Non-vegan:* "I don't really want to think about this right now. Can't we deal with it some other time?"
>
> *Vegan:* "I know this may be inconvenient for you, but we really need to figure this out. It'll make it easier in the future because we won't have to keep bringing it up."
>
> *Non-vegan:* "I guess so. But I don't want to have to think about it."
>
> *Vegan:* "That's ok. You don't have to! To make it easier, I can be the one in charge of buying groceries as long as you know that I'll only be bringing vegan food into the house."
>
> *Non-vegan:* "Fine. As long as it tastes good."

Even in the most difficult circumstances, remember that you have the right to speak up for what you believe in and be clear about your needs. This is not being demanding or picky or selfish. There is no need to apologize for living in alignment with your beliefs. It's also important to never compromise on those beliefs. Remember, you don't have to be a people pleaser. You're not responsible for other people's happiness, and it's not your responsibility to sacrifice your own needs to make someone else feel good. In my experience as an activist and educator, I've heard from many couples that the person who is vegan is expected to accommodate the non-vegan. Some scenarios include:

» Designating separate locations in the kitchen for vegan and non-vegan food;
» Cooking separate meals, one prepared by the vegan and one prepared by the non-vegan;
» Cooking a vegan meal that can be augmented by animal products;
» Accommodating the non-vegan by cooking meals with animal products at home

While these types of arrangements may satisfy the needs of the non-vegan, they infringe on the integrity of the vegan who must compromise his or her values to accommodate those who are not yet in sync with his or her ethics. This can offer short-term peace in the home, but it is illusory because it only puts off the inevitable. It is merely another facade that covers up a moral dilemma. Over time, the vegan's conscience becomes burdened with this inconsistency, and relationships may erode due to resentment over inauthenticity and complicity in contributing to unnecessary violence.

Instead of compromising one's values, the vegan has a moral obligation to demonstrate consistency in beliefs and actions. Saying "I can't do that" or "that would compromise my values" are honest statements that assert one's boundaries. Recognize the non-vegan's reluctance by expressing appreciation for his or her understanding and to alleviate any feelings of being forced to change. *"I realize this is a difficult adjustment for you, but we can make it work. You may even enjoy trying new foods!"*

Learning to say "No" is a difficult skill for the vegan to master. It means standing your ground and staying firm in your convictions. Think of it as confronting a status quo that is based on oppression and exploitation, rather than confronting any one individual. When you say "No," you are not dismissing the objections of non-vegans so much as you're negating a culture that considers unnecessary violence and suffering normal. We must be clear in this fact and emphasize the distinction between the two. The non-vegan is defending what he or she has been conditioned to believe is indisputable reality: that meat is the only way to get protein, milk is for strong bones, vegans are weak, and many other misconceptions that will be explored further in the next chapter. These myths are difficult to overcome. That is why we must be honest and direct in our communication, firm in our convictions, and empathetic to those who have not yet been enlightened.

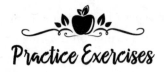

Practice Exercises

It takes courage to stand up for our beliefs, particularly when people we care about are not yet motivated to do the same. Through practice, we learn the gentle art of being assertive in conversations while also being respectful, honest, and kind. The following exercises help us develop those skills.

SELF-REFLECTION
Reflect on some difficult conversations you've had regarding your veganism and think about what went wrong. What do you want future conversations to look like? What can you do differently to make conversations more productive?

How can you be proactive in setting ground rules in your relationships?

VISUALIZATION
Describe your ideal living situation. What would that look like? How do you envision relationships with non-vegan family and friends? Imagine them as pre-vegans who are beginning to grasp the moral imperative of being vegan.

Chapter 3

Overcoming Obstacles

Wouldn't it be nice if all of our family and friends suddenly became vegan in solidarity with us and for the animals? Some of us are that fortunate, but for the rest of us, maintaining relationships with non-vegans is often our greatest ongoing challenge. We can be positive and encouraging and persistent in our convictions, and over time some non-vegans may become more receptive to the idea of changing their habits, but the truth of the matter is there are many psychological barriers and social saboteurs that interfere with our efforts. In this chapter we will explore the various myths and misconceptions people hold about veganism, assess an individual's readiness to change, and determine how best to focus your message to guide someone to take concrete steps that lead to living true to their values.

We need to keep in mind that we are making progress in every conversation we have, despite the reality that advocating for justice can be a long and difficult journey. Ida B. Wells-Barnett, who was the daughter of slaves, went on to become a journalist and co-founder of the National Association for the Advancement of Colored People (NAACP) in 1909. She was integral in fighting to overturn the repressive Jim Crow Laws, and refused to sit in the black section of a railroad car in Memphis, Tennessee, after paying for a first class ticket in the white "Ladies Section." Her words remind us that in seeking justice, we have an obligation to enlighten others. "The way to right wrongs is to turn the light of truth upon them." We must be the beacon in the lighthouse that guides those who may otherwise be lost.

Vegan Myth Busting

Anyone who's been vegan for longer than 5 minutes has undoubtedly been asked, "where do you get your protein?" In fact, it's probably one of the questions we wondered ourselves in the beginning. To be sure, we've done the research. There are numerous resources available on vegan nutrition to ensure that anyone can be healthy as long as they eat a wide variety of fresh fruits and vegetables, whole grains, beans, nuts, and seeds. All plant-based foods contain protein, and very little is needed to maintain optimal physiological functioning. While I won't get into an in-depth response to each of these myths, I will provide guidance for how to interpret each comment, analyze the person's motives, and frame an appropriate response with a question that redirects the focus of the conversation back to encouraging self-examination and reflecting on one's habits. A resource list to consult for further information can be found in the Appendix.

When you find yourself engaged in a potentially contentious conversation, take a moment to inhale deeply, visualize a positive outcome, and make an effort to use non-verbal cues such as eye contact, nodding your head in agreement, and leaning forward (as appropriate). Your ability to stay calm and focused will add to your credibility. Always remember that your goal is to educate the other person, not win an argument. It doesn't matter if you're "right" when the other person is unwilling to accept the information you are sharing. Instead, it's absolutely critical to establish a tone of trust and non-judgment. This can be achieved by using what's known as the "Socratic Method," a technique for engaging another person fully by asking questions and drawing out underlying ideas and presumptions. By responding to a question with another question, you are able to take charge of the conversation and remove any feeling of defensiveness. This also focuses the inquiry on self-examination and critical thinking where more profound insights may be gained. People are more likely to change when they are persuaded by emotion, because we often make decisions based on our feelings rather than facts. Gaining trust and connecting through personal stories builds that emotional foundation. Following are some common scenarios and strategies for addressing them.

> **Vegan food is boring:** While it would be easy to quickly retort, "No, it's not!" such a knee-jerk response would curtail continued dialogue. Instead, invite self-reflection by responding with a question, such as, "why do you think it's boring?" The person may answer by saying, "all you can eat are salads." Acknowledge this concern, but refrain from correcting. "Yes, it's true that vegans eat salads, but there are so many more types of meals we can eat. What kinds of food do you like?" Asking another question invites the person to again do some thinking, and this time it gets them to disclose their taste preferences. Once you know that, you can respond by saying, "all of the foods you just described can

easily be 'veganized,' and you'd enjoy them just as much. Plus, they're much healthier for you and no animals had to suffer for your enjoyment."

It's so expensive!: This comment addresses an underlying concern that a person needs to shop at specialty grocery stores to be vegan and that doing so is dramatically different from their usual routine, which would make it prohibitive for them. It's also an indication of the mistaken belief that vegan food is inaccessible, which can be a factor for someone without the financial means or ability to shop outside of his or her own neighborhood. Indeed, food deserts make shopping for fresh fruits and vegetables difficult. Acknowledge that concern, then turn your response around by asking a question: "You're right. It *can* be expensive if you choose to shop at specialty grocery stores, but fortunately there are many affordable alternatives available at regular supermarkets, discount chains like Walmart, and convenience stores like 7-Eleven. Even farmers markets provide low-cost options. Where do you usually shop for food?" After the person states where they shop, indicate that vegan staples such as rice and beans, pasta, nut butters, fruits, and veggies can be found there and that most major grocery stores even have "natural foods" sections stocked with plant-based meat and dairy alternatives that are oftentimes less expensive than animal products. For those on a limited budget, many farmers markets across the United States accept Supplemental Nutrition Assistance Program (SNAP) and FMNP (Farmers' Market Nutrition Program) for the purchase of fresh fruits and vegetables. SNAP benefits can even be doubled with the Double Dollars program at participating farmers markets. (For a list of farmers markets that accept SNAP see www.fns.usda.gov/ebt/snap-and-farmers-markets) Other cost-saving tips include buying in bulk, shopping for "seconds" in the not so pretty produce section, buying local produce when it's in season, and going to discount stores such as Ocean State Job Lot and home goods stores like Marshall's and TJMaxx for pantry staples. Let them know it's easy to stretch your dollars as a vegan if you're a smart shopper.

Too many carbs!: The misconception here is that vegan food is loaded with carbs and that it's unhealthy. While we know that carbohydrates are an essential macronutrient, many people mistakenly believe that they cause weight gain and lead to obesity. It's important to clarify that refined carbohydrates stripped of any nutritive value are indeed unhealthy if consumed on a regular basis; however, whole plant-based foods in their natural state contain fiber, antioxidants, vitamins, and minerals which are essential to our health. One response might be to say, "did you know that most plant-based foods contain the perfect ratio of carbohydrate-protein-fat (65%-25%-10%) for optimal energy efficiency? What kinds of foods do you eat that are equally efficient?" A followup to that question might be the myth that animal products are necessary for protein (see below).

I'm Paleo, and I need my meat: After agreeing that it's good to eat a more natural diet by eliminating processed foods, junk food and sugar sweetened beverages, you can inquire, "why do you think you need to eat animal flesh?" It's a common misconception that the only way to get complete protein and iron in our diet is by eating meat. Fortunately, you can explain that there are numerous plant-based food sources that contain all nine essential amino acids the body can't produce, including hemp seed, chia seed, soy, quinoa, spirulina, nutritional yeast, amaranth, and buckwheat. It's also important to note that eating a wide variety of plant-based foods can ensure consuming all the necessary amino acids over the course of a day and that they don't need to be combined in one meal. Ask the person, "do you know how to prevent iron deficiency?" Explain that iron is easily obtained through plant-based sources such as dried fruits, beans and lentils, whole grains, dark leafy green vegetables like kale and collard, tofu, and tempeh. The problem is not that vegans don't get enough iron in their diet, but in order to increase iron absorption these foods must be consumed with foods containing vitamin C. Usually adding dark leafy greens or a squeeze of lemon to the meal takes care of that easily. This is important even for non-vegans.

Rabbit food. Twigs and berries. It's just weird: There are any number of dismissive responses that you will hear from people who are too closed-minded and unwilling to listen to what you have to say. These are defense mechanisms that attempt to block out new ways of thinking. It's important to recognize them for what they are and not become frustrated attempting to overcome them. Not everyone is respectful, nor are they genuinely interested in learning about veganism, and that's ok. While we might wish that everyone cared as much about this as we do, accept that many people don't, at least initially. It's also good to remember that no matter how effective we are as communicators and as noble as our intentions are, we can't change everyone. Even more important, we shouldn't get attached to results. By that I mean we cannot "make" someone go vegan, and we're not failures if they don't. We need to remain positive no matter what the outcome of each conversation may be, simply for the fact that we have spoken up and shared our truth.

So, what do we do with the defensive brush-off? Depending on our relationship with the person, one approach might be to inject some humor that might point out the absurdity of the comment, such as:

> *"It's rabbit food"*
> *"Hey, cool. Rabbit Food would be a great name for a restaurant. Thanks for the idea!"*
>
> *"Twigs and berries"*
> *"Good point! When we're lost in the forest together I'll be able to survive on twigs and berries while you're out foraging for hamburgers. Awesome!"*
>
> *"It's just weird"*
> *"Well ya know, like the bumper sticker says, "Why be normal?""*

Another approach, particularly if you sense that the conversation has potential to get derailed by ad hominem attacks, is to thank the person for considering veganism and refer them to a website, documentary, or other resource for additional information. Some good ones can be found in the Appendix at the end of this book. For your own practice, I recommend familiarizing yourself with detailed responses to common concerns such as these by studying the following books:

> » *Eat Like You Care* by Gary Francione and Anna Charlton
> » *Mind If I Order the Cheeseburger* by Sherry Kolb
> » *Becoming Vegan* by Brenda Davis, RD and Vesanto Melina, RD

Are You Ready?

Conversations such as these are good indicators of a person's readiness to change. The fact that someone is willing to engage with you in this manner is an encouraging first step. How else will they learn of the many positive reasons for being vegan? Further, the kinds of questions they ask as well as their ability to reflect on your responses should indicate to you if they are open to these ideas or simply giving lip service to them. When I first went vegan I didn't have all of the answers — none of us do — and I felt hesitant to initiate discussions because I was afraid of getting stumped by a tricky question. Since then, I've learned that it doesn't matter if we're not experts; what matters most is our ability to tell our story and to be able to recognize that our actions have consequences, many of which are hidden from us. We may not ever know that a 5-minute conversation we had with someone a year ago was the turning point in their life that lead them to become vegan, as well as a more engaged person within their community. This is the message to share. I can confirm this to be true after being stopped while grocery shopping by someone who came running over to tell me she had attended one of my cooking demos 7 years prior and after following my recommendation to go vegan, her life completely changed (for the better!).

No matter how someone approaches us — whether confrontational or curious — it's important to make connections. Emphasize your similarities with the other person and open up the path to empathy with statements such as, "I never realized how animals were treated either, until I started doing some research." "I grew up eating animals' bodies, eggs, and milk, and thought it was normal, too." "When I learned that we don't need to eat animals to be healthy I was surprised, too. In fact, it made me pretty damn angry."

Many times, anger is the emotion that is stirred up, because no one wants to admit they've been lied to and that by not changing they remain complicit in the lie. Most people find it easier to look away rather than change behaviors. Our being vegan reminds them of the moral conflict lurking below the surface that they prefer to ignore. We're socialized since infancy to do what we're told, follow the example of our parents, and obey the rules for our own benefit. This is how we acculturate into the dominant system. The fact that the underlying system, which establishes what's acceptable and appropriate, is based on unnecessary violence and exploitation of non-human animals never enters our minds. It's a painful reality none of us wants to accept, but we must in order to change.

Move Into Your Discomfort Zone

One of the biggest obstacles to overcome is our own discomfort in social situations, particularly when it feels as if we're "the bad guy" when we speak up. This is a heavy burden to carry, and it's difficult to overcome at first. Be assured that the more you do it, the easier it becomes. Conversely, there are others who are so angered by what they've learned that every interaction with a non-vegan is filled with rage and hostility. While it's essential that we expose the truth, we need to remember that our ability to effectively communicate that truth with honesty and empathy will have the best chances of being heard. No one wants to be told they're a bad person.

I tend to be introspective by nature and non-confrontational in my daily life, but when I become aware of injustice, I feel compelled to expose it. But it isn't easy. For me, engaging in activism has given me confidence to speak up. Protesting at a circus, demonstrating against a pet store that sells animals obtained from puppy mills, leafletting on college campuses, holding vegan cooking demonstrations at public venues, and disrupting events where animals are being exploited are activities I've engaged in that, though uncomfortable at first, have left me feeling empowered. When joining with like-minded people who are motivated to educate the general public, collectively we become a force of change. That is a feeling to continue to hold onto even during the most difficult interactions.

I often think of the climax of the Dr. Seuss story, *Horton Hears a Who*, where the people of Whoville are all shouting in unison to save themselves, "We are HERE! We are HERE! WE ARE HERE!!!" We can do this if we stick together. Always remember: you are not alone.

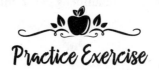

Practice Exercise

Confronting the status quo can be very stressful. As vegans, we do it every day simply by living in alignment with our beliefs. It's important to remind ourselves that being vegan is an act of courage that has potential for massive social change when we act together to disrupt a system of exploitation and violence. This can be very empowering personally as well as collectively, but we must always remember that with this power comes responsibility. It's up to us to be the catalyst for change.

POSITIVE AFFIRMATIONS

When interacting with non-vegans, imagine your conversation as a key opening a door. You are unlocking truth and inner wisdom. *(e.g.., "I am making a difference in the word," "I am speaking the truth," "No matter how hard this is, it's worth it," "My actions are helping animals.")*

VISUALIZATION

Each time you move into your discomfort zone, visualize outcomes and make statements that value your contributions. Describe the impact you want to have on those around you. *(e.g., "I am enabling this person to reconnect with her true nature that's based in compassion," "This conversation is a turning point in her life.")*

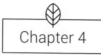

Chapter 4

Socializing

When I teach classes or give public presentations with audiences consisting primarily of non-vegans, one of the comments I hear most often after I'm finished is that they would be happy to go vegan if society was more accepting. Of course, my response to that is always, "we ARE society." What we do and how we act sets an example for others to follow. This is why it's so important to be proactive as a vegan while socializing.

Nonetheless, I get where they're coming from. The idea of being vegan may be unfamiliar to them and they're not aware of the wealth of resources available on the internet, from plant-based nutrition experts, on vegan retail sites, from plant-based meal delivery services, and within vegan communities, both in person and online. In short, they're hesitant to begin, because the idea of giving something up appears much more daunting in comparison to what they will gain. One of their biggest anxieties is the idea of not being able to carry on socializing with those who are not vegan, as was discussed in the previous chapters. The real risk of losing people close to us can sometimes feel more overwhelming than actually changing our diet. We've all encountered situations in which others just couldn't accept our veganism, for one reason or another, and that becomes an obstacle within the relationship. But we are living proof that it's possible to survive these losses. New connections are made within the growing global vegan community, and many of us often feel that the new friendships we develop are richer and much more rewarding than those that have drifted away. This is a natural part of being human and maturing into an enlightened adult. While it's incredibly fortunate to have friendships that last for decades and decades and grow as we do, very often our growth as individuals is reflected in the friendships we choose to cultivate during different periods in our life. We can encourage non-vegans by reassuring them that they will always have a network of friends when they connect with like-minded people who are supportive and respectful of their decision to live true to their values and beliefs. We expand our social circles by expanding our compassion and connection to people on a deeper level.

Hanging Out with Friends

Routine is tough to break, and when you look forward to the end of every workweek so you can kick back and enjoy a night out at your favorite restaurant with friends or co-workers, it's disconcerting to realize that nothing on the menu is vegan. This is the reality check many of us face when first becoming vegan, and it can be disillusioning. Our eyes are suddenly opened to the incredible amount of suffering contained in nearly every menu of every restaurant we're used to frequenting. We no longer feel comfortable supporting these establishments, but we're at a loss as to how to go about finding alternatives. The key here is to learn how to be assertive, creative, and adventurous with food.

Return to your list of Ground Rules that you established in Chapter 2. If you haven't already set some for yourself, now is the time to do so. It's important to consider your comfort level with friends as well as your authenticity as a vegan activist. Some questions to ask yourself include:

> » Will you frequent only vegetarian or vegan restaurants?
> » Order only vegan menu items at non-vegan restaurants while others order what they prefer?
> » Request non-vegans not order animal products?
> » Not dine where the bodies of animals are being served?
> » Request restaurants and food service establishments add vegan items to their menus?

I have personally chosen to follow each of these scenarios at different times depending on circumstances and company, with varying levels of success. Guiding each decision was feeling that my personal needs for authenticity were met and I was supporting the rights of animals while also educating others in a non-confrontational way. I realize it's truly a juggling act to accomplish all three of these goals, and that's why I recommend frequent reflection and self-examination, ideally after each interaction we have with non-vegans.

In my early days as a vegan, I didn't want to disrupt my routine any more than I had to, nor did I want to inconvenience anyone. As a former "people pleaser," I often just went along where everyone else wanted to go and made do with a salad or French fries if the vegan offerings were limited. Or I brought food with me or ate ahead so that I didn't have to worry about going home hungry (and being cranky the whole time!). These are all adequate coping strategies, but they do little to educate, and they often leave the vegan feeling disempowered and frustrated.

As I gradually gained more confidence and began experimenting with new foods, I discovered it was simple to find vegan menu items at Japanese, Chinese, and Thai restaurants, and that Mexican and Indian staples like burritos and curries could easily be veganized by eliminating dairy products such as cheese, sour cream, ghee, yogurt, and cream. Even the old standby of pasta or chili can be found at most family style Italian-American restaurants. It also helps to call ahead and speak with the executive chef of a restaurant you plan to visit to request a vegan meal that's made from ingredients the restaurant has on hand. This is known as ordering "off menu," and many times chefs are happy to accommodate these requests since it gives them the opportunity to utilize their creativity. I've done this on such occasions as weddings and business events and have even been successful in getting restaurants to add vegan items to their regular menus. By incorporating vegan-friendly venues like these to your dining repertoire, you can encourage the adventurous members of your social circles to join you, perhaps with a goal of experimenting with a new restaurant each month. That way you can wean yourself off the old meat-centric establishments and discover exciting new dishes you and your friends can enjoy together. This can all be accomplished with little disruption to your usual socializing routine.

Dating While Vegan

Another challenging social situation many of us face is being single and seeking a partner who has compatible values. Here again we must each recognize our comfort level with interacting among non-vegans, which involves much deeper self-evaluation than simply setting the ground rules for dining out. The reality is that the pool of available vegans is limited. As such, we must determine what is acceptable to us in a dating partner by considering the following:

» Do we date only vegans? What about vegetarians?

» If we consider dating non-vegans, what ground rules are absolutely critical? And when do we discuss them with the other person... on or before the first date? Only after several weeks/months of dating? Only if we perceive there may be long-term compatibility?

» What requests do we make of a non-vegan dating partner regarding willingness to go vegan? Do we give a mandate to make the vegan transition? Do we set a time limit?

» Can we accept being in a relationship with someone who says that he or she "isn't ready" to make the vegan transition? What if they are *never* ready?

» And if our dating partners are unwilling to change their behaviors to be more in alignment with our lifestyle, do we choose to end the relationship and remain single instead of committing to a rigid non-vegan?

When I became vegan 20 years ago, I was married to someone I had known for nearly ten years. We were best friends and confided in each other completely. I explained to him that I needed to change my diet so that I could regain my health and so we could keep our beloved dog Lily, and he was understanding and 100% supportive. He agreed that my wellbeing was the number one priority. But when I also explained that one of the ground rules was that we maintain a vegan kitchen and that all meals we ate together be vegan, he was a little less enthusiastic. It didn't make sense to him that he should have to change as well, and he understandably felt imposed upon. Nonetheless, I persevered. I was in a health crisis that needed my strict adherence to plant-based whole foods; as a recovering junk food addict I couldn't afford to have anything in the house that might sabotage my efforts. Even more so, once I became committed to ethical veganism, I couldn't bear the sight of animal body parts in the fridge next to my broccoli and tofu. So he agreed to eat vegan with me with one caveat: "as long as it tastes good." Thus, it was settled. Within 6 months I had regained my health and he had lost 50 pounds effortlessly. We both had more energy and stamina and started hiking together more frequently. He began riding his bike every day and in a year he was proud to say he was down to 185 lbs. and felt in better shape than when he was captain of his high school's cycling team.

This is what worked for our relationship at the time. I know of other vegans who make the vegan transition alone and resign themselves to tolerating their dating partner's meat eating. Some vegans have told me they don't even mention that they're vegan until the third or fourth date, and sometimes only when asked in a sort of "don't ask, don't tell" charade. One woman even told me, proudly, that her boyfriend thought she was just "on a diet" for a whole year. Although these tactics may have worked for them, they are hardly honest or authentic. Striking that balance can be difficult while dating. Since getting divorced and having been on many dates with non-vegans, I've been told that I have "impossibly high standards for anyone to live up to" (or at least too high for him), that I'm "too positive a person" (apparently he was only familiar with the angry militant vegan stereotype), and that "it would be too intimidating to be your boyfriend since you're smart, funny, pretty, kind, and an amazing chef" (with the implication that these qualities are too difficult to live up to and would leave the other person feeling inadequate).

I share these experiences to let you know that I'm aware of how difficult it is to find someone who understands and respects you, who values you for your ethical integrity, and who is similarly ethically inclined and worthy of your respect. I say this not to sound bleak, but rather, to emphasize that no matter who you date, your baseline should always be to remain true to yourself by being honest about your beliefs, assertive in stating your needs, and empathetic in understanding differences. And when those criteria aren't met, know that your convictions are far too important to ever settle for less. Jessica Ainscough was an advocate of alternative cancer treatments who went by the name The Wellness Warrior. Despite suffering from cancer as a child and later succumbing to the disease, she remained positive throughout her life, asserting, "Don't let someone dim your light simply because it's shining in their eyes." In dating as well as in any social situation, never be afraid to shine.

In the Workplace, School, and Other Organizations

We can run into some tricky situations when it comes to our workplaces. Some of us do business over meals with our co-workers and clients and we're often faced with the question of how to handle dining etiquette. If we are fortunate, we have a say in restaurant selection and can graciously make our needs known to the host. More often than not, the dining destination is a decision that is imposed upon us. Other times, when a meal is brought in for a meeting or other business event, it can be a challenge to get our needs met. To proactively manage these scenarios, I've found that it's best to inform your boss in advance that you're vegan in order to avoid any awkwardness that could impact business at a meeting. That way, you're making your needs known in advance and addressing any concerns in an assertive manner. Always have the view that responsible leadership recognizes others' needs and accommodates requests. Do not hesitate to express your needs in a respectful, thoughtful way. Let your boss know your ground rules for dining with co-workers, and thank him or her for their understanding. Wherever you go, start with a positive outlook and be supportive of any efforts to accommodate your needs. If you can speak to the chef in advance of your visit, offer to give him or her a list of foods you can/can't have to make it easier for them to plan. Your appreciation and enthusiasm can inspire the chef to get creative with the ingredients and make an outstanding meal that you will enjoy.

The same strategy can apply to an educational setting. Public school systems across the country have been mandated by the U.S. government to offer healthy and nutritious food to students. While this sounds promising, the reality is that healthy often means low-fat milk and chicken nuggets by the major dining services companies. We are gradually changing those definitions through various plant-based food initiatives in schools (e.g., NY Coalition for Healthy Food), and there is even an entirely vegan school in California (James Cameron and Suzy Amis' MUSE School in Calabasas). Many of the big animal welfare non-profits such as HSUS and PETA offer booklets for veganizing school cafeterias that can be shared with dining services directors. Some schools have adopted "Meatless Mondays" policies, and universities like UC San Diego even have entirely vegan dining halls. As always, the key to making these shifts is to be proactive and persistent, provide plenty of information, and always praise efforts to move in the vegan direction. See the Appendix for a list of resources.

Whether we belong to a church or synagogue, participate in a political party, or are members of a hobby group or civic organization, we often encounter difficulties dining among our peers. It can be a challenge at first, but by practicing the previously discussed techniques of setting ground rules and asserting your needs, you may find that you will soon be taking a leadership role in expanding not only vegan offerings, but the hearts and minds of your associates. Depending on the situation as well as your comfort level, this may also be an opportunity for education and outreach. Some vegans I know who are members of a Unitarian Universalist Church held a movie screening of the documentary "Cowspiracy" for their congregation followed by a discussion. This event lead to more interest to continue the conversation and a vegan potluck was organized. A core group continues to get together on a regular basis to expand the vegan message within their community, and they recently purchased a sermon on veganism at a church fundraiser. The pastor gave two sermons titled "Food Revolution" which introduced the entire congregation to the health benefits of a plant-based diet, the environmental degradation caused by animal agriculture, and the inherent cruelty and suffering of animals. Other possible outreach methods might include offering a presentation on veganism at a public school, hosting a vegan cooking class or potluck with guest speaker, sharing literature at events, tabling at church fairs, hosting a vegan bake sale fundraiser for an animal sanctuary, holding meetings at your home and providing vegan goodies, requesting donations to a farm animal rescue organization in lieu of birthday gifts, leaving vegan literature in your doctor's office (ask first!), or creating a vegan display in an office or at your public library. The possibilities are endless, but the key is to always think of how you can contribute to the benefit of your organization while also spreading the vegan message.

Traveling While Vegan

Ready for a road trip? I'm always game! Fortunately, websites such as Happy Cow (www.happycow.net) and Veg Dining (www.vegdining.com) make it easy for us vegan travelers to find oases across the country and around the world. I sometimes even plan vacations around locations that I know are vegan-friendly. Meccas such as San Francisco, Los Angeles, Portland, OR, Chicago, Austin, New York, Philadelphia, and Boston never fail to impress, and even smaller cities like Bethlehem, PA, Omaha, NB, Syracuse, NY, and Portland, ME offer hidden gems like decadent Vegan Treats, Isa Moskowitz's Modern Love, social justice in a vegan milk shake at Strong Hearts Cafe, and opportunities for vegan backwoods trailblazing on the northeastern shoreline through Maine Huts & Trails. I always find that the most difficult part is that there are too many places to eat, not enough time to get to all of them, and never enough room in my belly.

Nonetheless, I recognize that there are vast swaths of this country that are void of any dining establishments that cater to vegans. I've driven cross-country several times and learned a few tricks that kept me nourished and happy. The #1 rule is to live by the Boy Scout motto: "Always be prepared." I carry a bag filled with dry goods like nuts, seeds, dried fruit, and various packaged snacks to keep myself satisfied while driving 6-8 hours straight. Hydrating is also essential, so filling a cooler with fresh fruits and veggies when I leave home keeps me going, and I can always find something to grab-n-go when pit-stopping at local supermarkets and gas stations to restock the ice. I use these same strategies for air travel, but on a smaller scale. My carry-on bag doubles as a snack warehouse, because I never go far without a Larabar. Oranges and apples are also good portable snacks that provide some refreshment, and as far as I know, they're not on the TSA banned substance list.

Expanding Your Social Circles

When following these strategies, it's inevitable that your social circles will expand to include more like-minded people. Introducing non-vegan friends to veganism by participating in activities together such as attending vegfests, vegan cooking classes, and vegan health and nutrition lectures can expand their knowledge and pique their curiosity. Who doesn't like sampling yummy vegan goodies? We know the joy that practicing a vegan lifestyle brings, and when your loved ones are surrounded by others who share that passion, it's inevitable that some of it will rub off.

My mom has been my greatest success in this arena. When I started inviting her to join me at vegan cooking classes that I was teaching, she became curious, so I shared some literature and a few of my favorite cookbooks with her. The next thing I knew she was trying new recipes and sharing them with me. It became an adventure for both of us to share our passion for cooking together. Now she has become adept at veganizing family favorites, and I look forward to her super moist carrot cake with Tofutti cream cheese frosting every birthday (see Chapter 9). She likewise looks forward to attending events and reconnecting with friends she's made in the vegan community. We can all grow as a result of reaching out to people we love, by being inclusive rather than defensive, and sharing our passion and purpose with them so they can join us on this journey.

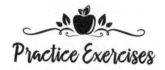

Practice Exercises

While it's tempting to resign yourself to believing your non-vegan friends and family will never become vegan, make a point of including them in your vegan activities. The more they feel welcomed, the less uncomfortable they will be in not only accepting your veganism, but also exploring it themselves. Give them plenty of opportunities to engage their curiosity so that they will be prompted to learn more on their own. Remember, it's not about forcing anyone to do anything they don't want to do, but rather stimulating their interest and being their helpful guide.

SETTING GOALS

What is your greatest frustration? Is it holiday dinners with family, an unsupportive workplace, friends who are hesitant to try something labeled vegan, or a significant other who just isn't ready to commit to veganism? List the Top 3 issues you'd like to resolve in your relationships that would help you to fully live a joyful vegan lifestyle.

ACTION STEPS

What can you do right now that will accomplish your goals of becoming an ambassador for veganism with non-vegan family and friends? What do you need from them to make this happen? Make a list of activities you can do with them to get the ball rolling *(eg. attend a cooking class together, cook a vegan meal for them, watch a vegan documentary together, let them choose a recipe from your favorite vegan cookbook for you to make, host a vegan potluck, etc.).*

POSITIVE AFFIRMATIONS

Envision yourself surrounded by supportive family and friends, in a welcoming workplace, and embraced by a community of like-minded people. Describe what your life would look and feel like once all the obstacles have been resolved *(e.g., "I have perfect relationships with family and friends who are no longer pre-vegans but fully fledged vegans. I enjoy their company so much more now that we can be authentic with each other and I am grateful for their understanding, love, and support.").*

Chapter 5

Becoming a Vegan Gardener

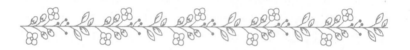

As an avid gardener, I'm very much in tune with the cycles of nature and what it takes for plants to thrive. Dedication, attention, patience, and lots of physical labor and TLC are the effort I put in that pay off with a bountiful harvest throughout the growing season. I apply these same principles to my vegan practice, equating my vegan community with an initially vacant patch of land that's been cultivated, tended, and nurtured in the same manner to yield an abundance of amazing friends. People are like plants in that they flourish when we give them attention. Some need more than others, and some may never grow, and we learn through experience where to focus our energy. From a Buddhist perspective, we also learn not to get attached to results, and that being mindful of the process is what matters most. So, even though we dream of lush and leafy plants that payoff with big fat juicy red heirloom tomatoes to slice up for our vegan grilled cheese sandwiches, we can't expect that every single crop will hit the motherlode. There are obstacles that get in the way that compete for our time and attention, and sometimes the unexpected occurs like drought and torrential rains. With both gardening and vegan activism, we learn through observation as well as trial and error how to face these challenges. What follows in this chapter is a guide for growing your own vegan community by using principles practiced by every good gardener.

Planting Seeds

Every day we have the opportunity to plant seeds simply by being positive vegan role models. In fact, this is one of the most effective methods for everyday activism. It may not necessarily reap instantaneous rewards or be easy to quantify, but each conversation we have, question we answer, recommendation we give, or resource we provide can be the necessary seed that will some day take root and grow. Much of gardening is about having faith, and the same is true for vegan activism. While we can't readily measure the effectiveness of our effort by directly attributing it to an immediate shift in behavior, there is indeed a correlation between what we say and do and whether our words are heard and heeded. Know that in widely scattering these seeds of compassion you are always increasing the chances that some will germinate.

I've probably given over a hundred presentations in the past 15 years of doing vegan activism. In that time I've had dozens of people tell me afterward they never realized how easy it was to be vegan and that they were going to give it a try. Even more rewarding is when people return to one of my events years later and tell me that my presentation changed their life. I love hearing stories of how a talk I gave or something I said triggered them to to do more research, to watch a documentary, to buy a vegan cookbook, to test a new recipe, or to make a simple change in their life that eventually lead them down the path to veganism. I once had a woman come running up to me after a presentation with tears in her eyes to say, "I just came here to tell you you saved my life 7 years ago!" I think we were both in tears after that.

Shining the Light of Truth

In addition to running my vegan personal chef business, I'm also a part-time faculty member at a community college in New Haven, Connecticut. Even though my job is to teach English, I always manage to find a way to weave veganism and other social justice issues into the lessons. I speak honestly and directly, often sharing information that my students tell me they've never heard before. "Why didn't somebody ever tell me this??!" they say incredulously. This is the common response for many of us when our eyes are first opened to the truth. Why have we been deceived? How can we just go on living like this once we know? It's all so impossible to fathom at first.

This is why it's always so important to spread the vegan message and never be afraid of shining the light on the truth. Like the escaped slave Sojourner Truth, who became an abolitionist and women's rights activist, once said, "Life is a hard battle anyway. If we laugh and sing a little as we fight the good fight of freedom, it makes it all go easier. I will not allow my life's light to be determined by the darkness around me." In this way we become beacons that guide those who are lost, confused, or stranded. We lift people up by encouraging them to recognize their inherent compassion for animals. We empower them to be true to their values so they can grow into the fully conscious human they were destined to become.

It's beyond exciting when a student asks me for more information or when, years later while walking through the halls, I bump into a former student who tells me he went vegan because of something I taught him. This is why I know every conversation matters. It is a rare instance when we receive confirmation that our everyday vegan activism had direct results. Nonetheless, always know that there are a multitude of others you will never hear from that you still may have managed to reach. Trust that you are making a difference in their lives.

Fertilize with the Right Nutrients

The tone with which we speak matters, and we should always reflect on the context as well as the content of our conversations. Do we want to shame someone for eating animals and their secretions, or do we want to help them see animals as individuals and extend their inherent empathy to all beings? Do we want to direct our anger and frustration at someone who does not yet understand their contribution to unnecessary violence, or do we want to help them realize their disconnection? When someone is not yet enlightened, it is up to those of us who are aware of the tremendous suffering of animals to be able to explain this reality in a non-judgmental way. For example, acknowledging that you were also once unaware of these issues can be the bridge that allows a difficult conversation with a non-vegan to continue. Remember where you came from before becoming vegan. No one likes finding out they're complicit in cruelty, particularly when they're not ready to disengage from practices that to them feel, to paraphrase Melanie Joy, natural, normal, and necessary.[1] Sharing your personal story of how you changed once you were confronted by that cognitive dissonance can create a path for them to follow. In some cases, it helps to have a simple one-line response ready for when someone asks the question, "Why are you vegan?" Make it personal, and let it speak for you.

> » I care about animals and don't want them to die for me.
> » I don't want to contribute to unnecessary suffering in the world.

---

1. See Melanie Joy's outstanding resource, *Why we love dogs, eat pigs, and wear cows: an introduction to carnism: the belief system that enables us to eat some animals and not others.* San Francisco: Conari Press, 2011.

- » I love animals and don't want to harm them.
- » I'm opposed to animal cruelty.
- » Everyone has an inherent right to live life on their own terms, including animals.
- » Animals are not ours to use.
- » Why are you not?

In the case of the last answer, remember that using the Socratic Method of responding to a question by asking another question not only takes attention off you, but more importantly, it encourages self-examination for the non-vegan. Rather than get into a tennis match where you're constantly volleying answers for every question the non-vegan slams at you, turn the conversation around and take control by being the one who asks the questions. I always recommend this technique particularly when a conversation has the potential to get heated and divisive. Instead of responding defensively with a sarcastic quip, it's always a good idea to take a moment to gather your thoughts, reflect on your emotions, and take a breath before formulating a question that gets at the heart of the matter. In many cases, the non-vegan feels threatened by the information you're presenting and he or she will bombard you with questions or accusations as a diversion tactic. It's important to recognize when this happens and not fall into that trap. You have an opportunity to make real headway if you address their concerns seriously and with full attention. Take charge, be assertive, and demonstrate confidence by engaging in honest, thoughtful dialogue. Below is an example of how the Socratic Method was used to guide a conversation that began with self-defeat and turned it into one of empowerment.

Non-vegan: "I could never be vegan."

Vegan: "Why do you think you could never be vegan?"

Non-vegan: "It's too hard."

Vegan: "What's the hardest thing about being vegan for you?"

Non-vegan: "I don't know. I just don't have the time to cook. I don't feel good when I try to eat vegan."

Vegan: "What kinds of vegan foods do you eat that make you not feel good?"

Non-vegan: "Well, it's not really that I don't feel good. It's just that I'm always hungry when I give up meat."

Vegan: "What kinds of food are you adding when you take away animal flesh?"

Non-vegan: "I'm not adding anything. I'm just eating less. And then I get hungry and tired."

Vegan: "Have you tried adding Gardein in place of the animal products? And eating more veggies??"

Non-vegan: "No. Huh. I guess I could do that. What's Gardein?"

Vegan: "Oh… you've never tried Gardein??! Well… let me tell you about it!"

Simple solutions to seemingly overwhelming obstacles can be reassuring to someone who is hesitant about even taking the first step to become vegan. When you take charge of the conversation, you can lead the non-vegan to these discoveries by rewiring their negative thinking patterns and demonstrating how open-minded curiosity can have positive results. This ensures them that the risk they're taking by changing something that is familiar is much better than following the same old habits that are unhealthy for themselves, other people, animals, and the planet.

Water Those Who Are Wilting

Despite all of our positive efforts, there are times when we encounter roadblocks that even the most effective communicator among us has trouble breaking through. It can be incredibly frustrating when your best attempts at connecting with someone make zero headway. Even worse, you find yourself becoming agitated by the non-vegan's lack of understanding or unwillingness to engage his or her own empathy towards animals. Whether it's a face to face conversation or a comment on a Facebook thread, we all can relate to the experience. We feel ineffective as vegan role models and want to give up. We feel hopeless that the world will never be vegan. We see only negativity around us and fall into the trap of believing the world is an ugly place. We curse all of humanity. When you find yourself descending into this kind of despair or see other vegans whose spirit has been crushed, remind each other that it's only temporary. It's a tough job to be always swimming against the tide of social norms and conformity, but you're doing it. And every vegan in the world is supporting you.

Weed Out Pests and Toxic Invaders

All of us have had those bad days. Sometimes we dread interactions with certain people because we know they always, inevitably, degenerate into unproductive conversations that drain us. We avoid these people and cringe when we see them. We obsess over the idea that we'll never get through to them. And in some cases, we may be right. It's important in these instances to accept that we can't have a positive impact on everyone, no matter what we do. But not only that, if we find that these scenarios become regular occurrences, we must recognize that it's time for some serious self-evaluation as well. What is it about them that triggers our own negativity? Why do we allow them to get under our skin and prevent us from having a productive interaction? Could it be that in the process of speaking up for animals we are also speaking up for ourselves and becoming personally invested in winning an argument? In Melanie Joy's excellent TED Talk, "Understanding Carnism for Effective Vegan Advocacy" (ARC 2016), she states that the goal of effective vegan advocacy is not to be right, not to win, and not to change someone. Our goal is to be understood, and to understand the other. To test that theory, ask yourself if your being right and getting the other person to admit they're wrong is more important than letting them figure it out for themselves. Or conversely, are they trying to convince you to question your own already examined convictions? In these cases where our ego becomes involved, we need to consciously make an effort to remove ourselves from the conversation so that it doesn't become personal. We need to weed out our own negative thoughts and judgments about other people and accept that they are not yet ready to absorb what we have to offer. Similarly, we may also need to consider the impact others have on our own mental health. If we are constantly doing battle with the same few people who diminish our energy reserves for educating others, we may need to make the decision to weed out those people from our lives who are toxic to our wellbeing. It's impossible to be an effective activist if we are constantly in a state of stress. Always be vigilant: pull out the weeds so you can make room for healthy plants to grow.

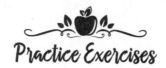

Practice Exercises

This chapter may lead you to make some difficult decisions. It's important to keep in mind the kind of garden you want to grow. If you want strong, healthy plants, you must nurture them every day, work hard, be patient and persistent, and have faith that in time your efforts will come to fruition. Don't let the weeds take over.

POSITIVE AFFIRMATIONS

Envision the world you are creating by being a positive vegan role model. Know that you are making a difference every day in all that you do. Think of how you nurture your vegan community and expand your circles to include non-vegan family and friends (*e.g., "I am surrounded by friends and family who are open-minded and supportive of my vegan lifestyle. I am creating the world I want to live in."*).

VISUALIZATION

What is your mission? Write it here and repeat it to yourself daily, and feel the effect it has on you as you begin to actualize it. What is your purpose? Write what you hope to achieve as a vegan activist. Remind yourself to recall these thoughts and feelings during challenging times.

My Mission:

My Purpose:

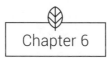

Chapter 6

Self-care for the Vegan Activist

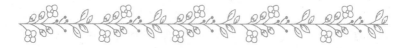

Throughout this book at the end of each chapter you've been given practice exercises which ask you to focus on setting goals, creating action steps to achieve them, visualizing outcomes, and stating positive affirmations that encompass what you want to see happen not only in your own life as a vegan activist, but in the world. These are techniques that train the mind to think positively and holistically by fostering a state of consciousness that is open to possibilities. Through these exercises we develop an unwavering belief that when we focus our efforts, we can achieve tremendous results. Nothing is impossible. I always tell my students that the only difference between success and failure is not giving up. This resilience and determination is absolutely essential to vegan activism. I hope you have found these exercises beneficial to your interactions with non-vegans.

Nonetheless, there are times when even our best efforts fall short of achieving our goals, and in those instances we must remind ourselves that self-compassion is of the highest priority. Stress reduction techniques such as meditation, yoga, qigong, tai chi, breathing exercises, and other forms of relaxation train the mind to stay positive and focused. The reality is that it can be difficult to remain optimistic amidst daily challenges and set-backs. We may become overwhelmed by the negativity around us and feel that our efforts are making little headway in ending it. We feel engulfed by a sea of apathy. We think the bad guys are winning. The curtain of sadness that falls down upon us may at times be too much to bear. While the temptation is to give up and retreat into our safe little cocoons, we know that remaining there would limit our effectiveness as vegan activists. The aware-ness of our own limitations can also lead to pangs of guilt and shame which further diminish our ability to help not only ani-mals, but ourselves. It's important to recognize when you reach these moments of crisis so that you can take a step back and reflect on your own well-being. What follows in this chapter is a series of strategies that will help you address self-care as a vegan activist — physically, mentally, and emotionally — so that you can remain a positive force for animals, people, and the planet.

Staying Focused

Compassion is absolutely essential when it comes to vegan activism. Sure, most of us find it easy to express our love of animals, and we wish everyone felt the same way as we do. But before we can recognize that capacity in others, we need to nurture our compassion for ourselves. Generosity, selflessness, and kindness are all positive qualities, but if we give so much that our energy is depleted, we may not have reserves left to take care of ourselves, and our health can suffer as a result. That in turn can negatively impact our ability to help others.

I have known many vegan activists who devote their lives to protecting animals. They are the ones who go out every morn-ing and evening to care for their feral cat colonies, in rain or snow, whether they're tired, hungry, or cold themselves. They sacrifice their own well-being in order to help those in need. They hold fundraisers and tag sales to raise money to pay for cat food and medical bills. They foster animals no one else will take in. They walk dogs at the local pound, table at events, volunteer at vegan festivals, carry signs at protests, and post petition after petition on the internet hoping others will care at least a fraction as much as they do. Before they know it, they are so caught up with the endless cycle of responding to emergencies that they are in perpetual crisis mode themselves. Who else will do it if not them? Just as one catastrophe is averted, another equally urgent situation appears which consumes their attention.

With adrenaline levels continuously spiked, it's nearly impossible to even take a moment to breathe. And yet, concentrating on one's breath is exactly what will help return peace and balance to these chaotic situations because it returns our mental focus to our own well-being. I've learned through over a decade of meditation practice that deep, meditative breathing exercises are the remedy to scattered thinking, confusion, and poor decision making. Focusing on one's breath centers the mind and directs energy toward positive thoughts. It's a method that forces a moment to slow down for self-reflection:

> *(breathe in deeply)* Am I doing what's best?
> *(breathe out fully)* Is this healthy?
>
> *(breathe in deeply)* Does this feel right?
> *(breathe out fully)* Can I ask for help?
>
> *(breathe in deeply)* Am I taking care of myself first?
> *(breathe out fully)* Reflect. Repeat.

Make no mistake, there will *always* be emergencies whether you've rescued one dog or one thousand. Yes, as activists we always wish we could save them all, and our efforts certainly have made a difference in many animals' lives. But we also must be mindful of self-care as a priority. Making this mental shift will help you become a positive role model for family and friends who will see that you put your beliefs into practice not only for animals, but for yourself. They care about you and want you to be healthy. No one expects you to be a martyr. When you demonstrate the ability to stay calm amidst chaos, you will not only become more effective as an activist, but you will inspire others to follow your lead.

Debriefing

After every conversation or situation which tests your abilities as a vegan activist, it's important to take some time to reflect on your effectiveness. The practice of asking yourself what worked and what didn't will help you develop skills as a powerful communicator in even the trickiest of circumstances. I do this every time I teach an English class, give a cooking lesson, participate in a protest, have a conversation about veganism, or present a lecture to hundreds of people. I want to know whether my message resonated with my audience. I can see it as well as feel it through the responses I receive. Sometimes it's in the eye contact I make with individuals who appear engaged and focused on my words. Other times it's in the questions they ask afterwards that demonstrate their curiosity has been piqued and there's an interest in learning more. If my words fall flat, if there's fidgeting, fussing, or worse, dead silence, I know I need to examine my presentation content as well as delivery. Knowing my audience's needs and whether or not I filled them is the first place I look. This is a technique popular in business as well as in Zen Buddhist practice. Geshe Michael Roach's classic book, *The Diamond Cutter: The Buddha on Managing Your Business and Your Life*, explores this concept though stories about the meticulous work of a diamond cutter who puts Buddhist principles into practice in his daily routine.[1] He develops a habit of introspection by paying attention to the details and maintaining integrity in his craft in order to achieve his client's expectations. This allows his true nature of kindness and generosity to emerge, even with the most unreasonable and demanding customer. Using this technique increases our effectiveness as everyday vegan activists, where we're always learning, always improving.

Periodically, it's beneficial to step back from your vegan activism to reflect on your effectiveness. This can be done not only after a situation that went poorly, but also when you find yourself making progress with those who previously seemed impossible to reach. It can shed light on whether a new communication strategy was successful, or if it was merely a change in circumstance that resulted in your favor. Conversely, when you reflect on frustrating conversations, you can determine what went wrong and how you can adjust your behavior in the future in order to prevent it from happening again. These are all learning experiences that are helping you become a better vegan activist, and it's only through conscious reflection and self-examination that you improve. We are less likely to be offended by adversarial comments or take them as personal attacks when we see them as opportunities to learn about ourselves and each other. Communication is an interactive process, and we need to focus on conveying our message with confidence, honesty, and kindness. It's not about winning an argument or proving someone is wrong.

Managing Burnout

When conversations become heated arguments that leave us feeling drained and demoralized, we need to step away. Inevitably there will be people who attempt to push our buttons, and if we respond with knee-jerk reactions, sarcasm, or other defense

1.Roach, Michael, and Christie McNally. *The diamond cutter: the Buddha on managing your business and your life.* New York: Doubleday, 2009.

mechanisms, we only feed the negativity that acts as a barrier to real behavior change. We are missing a critical piece of the communication process that leads to growth when we neglect to reflect and instead jump to hasty judgments. Once we become aware of the people and topics that trigger these emotional reactions in us, we can be more mindful in our responses and mentally prepare to let them go.

We also can't expect everyone will become vegan as a result of our interventions, at least not right away. This does not mean we give up, however. Instead, it's a matter of reframing our activism with more realistic expectations. Always remember that you are planting seeds with each positive conversation.

But I understand, through personal experience, that we can easily become engulfed in hopelessness when the negativity around us feels insurmountable. Often it's because we are either dwelling on past difficulties or worrying about what *could* happen in the future while also looping endless catastrophic scenarios in our minds that leave us numb. We dread seeing that family member who always seems ready to start an argument. Or we fret over the millions of animals dying every day whose lives we have little control over. Or maybe it's the latest animal cruelty investigation or abused animal photo circulating on Facebook that throws us into a tailspin. Whatever the cause, we find ourselves thinking, "It's never going to end," or "The world will never be vegan in my lifetime." While it's important to be realistic in our activism and aware of these issues, when our minds focus on the vast problems that exist in our society, we become a conduit for more negativity rather than a catalyst for change. Make a conscious effort to stop yourself from getting caught up in this endless cycle of despair. It's debilitating. Incessant brooding and commiserating only reinforces a sense of disempowerment that leads to an atmosphere of futility. When you find yourself stuck in this behavior pattern, take the time you need to disengage, recover, and regain your strength before returning to any activism.

Distance yourself from difficult people and take a break from social media.

The Dalai Lama presents a compelling case for managing this burden by being compassionate toward oneself and all beings. "No matter what is going on, never give up. Develop the heart. Too much energy... is spent on developing the mind instead of the heart. Be compassionate. Not just to your friends, but to everyone. Be compassionate. Work for peace in your heart and in the world. Work for peace. And I say again, never give up. No matter what is happening, no matter what is going on around you, never give up."

There are two rules to always remember.

1. To prevent burnout: have compassion for yourself.
2. To recover from burnout: have compassion for yourself.

Take a break and explore Mother Nature with a hike in the woods, a walk on the beach, or a drive to the mountains. Connect with animals by visiting a dog park, volunteering at an animal rescue organization, greeting animals at a farm sanctuary, or simply cuddling with your dog or cat or other companion animal. Get creative by drawing, painting, singing, or playing a music instrument. Dig in your garden. Mow the lawn. Plant a tree. Go to a movie. Read a book. Do whatever it takes to rekindle that joy for your amazing life and reconnect with your reasons for being the beautiful person you are.

Maintaining Inner Balance

Developing a mindfulness practice of meditation, yoga, qigong, tai chi, or other calming exercise is important for maintaining inner peace and balance. Not only will it help with managing burnout, but it will enable you to remain calm and focused during even the most difficult circumstances, as well as more resilient afterward. I began practicing meditation on a daily basis around 2001 while going through a divorce, and shortly after that I also incorporated yoga into my daily routine. Like nearly everyone who attempts meditation for the first time, I said I could never do it because my mind was always spinning with thoughts and worries, and my emotional state was clouded with so much anger, frustration, and grief. Not surprisingly, I was terrible at it at first. The physical discomfort of sitting for a mere 15 minutes straight combined with doing *nothing* was so foreign to me that I wanted to give up. Fortunately, I was taking a 15-week class so I decided to stick with it, and by the end of the semester I was hooked. Not only did I understand the concept of focused breathing, but I felt it having a positive effect on me physically, emotionally, and mentally. With each long inhale and exhale, I could feel the tension releasing from my body. My mind became clearer and less distracted. I no longer looped that negative script over and over in my head during moments of quiet. Instead, I was just quiet. I learned to accept the emptiness of loss and how to be in the present moment. Essentially, I was rewiring my brain. Below are some tips for achieving inner balance and overcoming adversity.

A daily practice of self-care is essential for the vegan activist. I begin each morning with meditation, breathing exercises, and yoga stretches that center and ground me. I think about activities I have planned for the day and repeat positive affirmations like a mantra which set my intentions. I return to these thoughts throughout the day and make a conscious effort to inhale deeply and exhale fully when feeling stressed, anxious, or rushed. These are some of the methods I've used through various times in my life when I've become engulfed in the depths of burnout:

> **Journaling:** When your mind is bogged down by debilitating thoughts, it's difficult sometimes to

even think straight. Keeping a journal where you can unload toxic thoughts helps break the pattern of futility. If you have trouble falling asleep because your mind can't stop spinning, write it down. Stream of consciousness purges like these are incredibly cleansing. Another time to write is first thing in the morning. Focus on whatever comes to mind: your plans for the day, obstacles you will face, positive affirmations, what makes you happy. Just write and let it flow. This is a mental workout that helps strengthen clarity of thought and remove judgments and other limitations to effective communication.

Drawing (or singing, painting, playing a musical instrument, or any other creative endeavor): Similar to writing, this is the process of unloading our mental burdens, but with a creative twist. I like to get a big box of crayons, choose whatever color appeals to me, and just start dragging the tip around the page of a sketch pad making abstract swirls and lines using various pressures to suit my emotional state. Sometimes they start off jagged and harsh with bits of crayon breaking off here and there; other times the colors flow together creating harmonious patterns that are pleasing to look at and ease my mind. No one needs to see these drawings but you. You don't have to be an artist or know anything about composition, perspective, or technique. Just let the crayons speak for you.

Gardening: Getting my hands dirty is one of the pleasures of gardening, along with the payoff of delicious veggies, of course. There's even evidence that soil bacteria on our skin improves mood and alleviates depression.[2] I enjoy the workout of digging in dirt and pulling out weeds, quenching thirsty plants with a soothing spray from the garden hose, and watching all of the activity from birds, bees, butterflies, and other insects who are part of my garden community. All of this alleviates stress and empties my mind of worries that accumulated through the day.

Connecting to Nature: Whether it's a 2-hour hike through a state forest, camping in the mountains, a stroll through a rose garden, or a walk on the beach while listening to waves and seagulls, when we connect with nature, we nurture our souls. If you're feeling depleted, look to Mother Nature for comfort and restoration.

Interacting with Animals: Needless to say, most of us are on our vegan journey because we love animals. Visiting a farmed animal sanctuary to meet and get to know the lucky few survivors can be not only enlightening but empowering, as they are evidence that what we do matters. On a local level, we can volunteer with animal rescue organizations by walking dogs and cuddling kitties, or foster if we're able. Sometimes even just going to the local dog park and watching the goofy delight of unbridled pooches in action can lift our spirits. I am fortunate to have shared my home with dogs and a cat who have brought me joy on the darkest days, and I depend on them for strength and resiliency.

---

2. Kennedy, Pagan. *How to Get High on Soil*, The Atlantic, January 31, 2012.

Retreating: Having a purpose in life is absolutely essential, but the desire to be needed and feeling that people can't live without us can sometimes become an unhealthy addiction if we don't take care of ourselves first. I highly recommend taking a mental health retreat for yourself (an overnight somewhere peaceful), to be able to separate from the demands of your life and appreciate just being alive. Once you come back, remember that experience whenever you get stressed out and sense the waves of burnout approaching.

We need to remember that, like other animals, we exist for our own reasons and do not belong to anyone else. Although we may have adult responsibilities, we must never allow them to control us and take away our freedom. Always know that you are making a difference in the world. Focus on the good you and others are doing and the many animals you've helped. Love and protect this planet with all your heart. Be grateful for every moment that you're alive. If the indifference and negativity of other people threaten your peace of mind, step away, let them go, and accept that they are not yet enlightened. Then continue to do everything you do to make the world a better place. You matter.

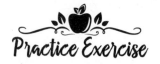

Practice Exercise

Always be mindful that you are making a difference in the world simply by being vegan. Focus your thoughts on the world you are creating: one that is kind, compassionate, and based on freedom and justice for all beings. Know your vision and embrace it as if everyone is already living it. This may seem naive and idealistic at first, but in practice it becomes a powerful demonstration of personal fortitude. YOU are setting the tone. YOU control how you see yourself. YOU decide what to accept. No one can take away this vision unless you let them.

POSITIVE AFFIRMATIONS

Focus on your strength and what you do best. Think of how you inspire others to share your vision of a vegan community. No matter what happens around you, even under the most difficult circumstances, you will be able to handle it. *(e.g., "I am strong, focused, grounded, and confident. I welcome whatever the universe sends me.")*

Repeat these statements to yourself whenever you question your ability as an activist or feel the burden of burnout holding you back.

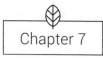

Chapter 7

Dress for Success

Now that you've sufficiently prepared yourself to handle any scenario that may arise within your non-vegan circles, it's time to have some fun! This is what we look forward to: the chance to play with food. Keep the joy of sharing good food as your guiding principle whenever you cook, and your passion for veganism will be contagious. For more than a decade running my vegan personal chef business, I've been fortunate to hear countless non-vegan clients exclaim with astonishment, "I never knew vegan food could be this good!" It's always rewarding to receive validation of what we already know, because it means someone is willing to open their mind to something they may have previously never believed was possible. Tantalize them with some delectable vegan treats, encourage them to come back for more, show them how easy it is to make the transition, and pretty soon you'll have a budding vegan in your life.

I often refer to people like this as "pre-vegans," because they're willing to move in the vegan direction and just need a little guidance to succeed. That's where this chapter is vital. You will learn strategies that have worked for me in my outreach among non-vegans, as well as practical ideas for establishing the right tone at the dinner table, creating menus that are inviting, taking the familiar and making it fabulous, and tips for staying positive, poised, and passionate in your vegan convictions. I'll also address the importance of mindful eating as a tool for engaging conscious compassion and overcoming obstacles with picky eaters.

First Impressions with Food

The food on our plates is a representation of our belief systems, a complex tapestry of our cultural heritage, socio-economic status, geography, ethical and moral convictions, and personal taste preferences. We make choices based on these factors every time we sit down to eat. Aside from restrictions of cost and convenience, the food we tend to prefer is visually appealing, tasty, and satisfying. Essentially, we want it to taste as good as it looks. In addition, we experience what Pamela Goyan Kittler calls the "Omnivore's Paradox," the contrast between a desire to explore new taste sensations but also stick with what's safe and familiar.[1] This paradox is what often is a challenge to non-vegans who may be curious to experiment with vegan food, but also hesitant because it is different. We can act as a vegan guide, serving as an indispensable resource for them as they navigate this unknown territory.

We've all heard the expression "you eat with your eyes," and this is particularly true when it comes to vegan food. There is a common misconception that vegan food is bland, boring, and beige. Instead, by seeing cooking as an adventure and creating a veritable rainbow on your plate, you can overcome any hesitancy among non-vegans. We create positive first impressions by presenting food that someone can't wait to dig into.

1.Kittler, P. G., Sucher, K. P., & Nahikian-Nelms, M. (2011). *Food and Culture*. USA: Wadsworth.

Setting the Table

There are several guidelines I follow as a chef in order to elicit eager enthusiasm from non-vegans. This is how I set the table for success. It's not literally about having the perfect place settings of fine china and polished silverware, although that can be a nice accoutrement. Instead, it's a matter of creating an atmosphere of adventure and curiosity where guests are encouraged to experiment, tempered with familiarity and comfort to help overcome any hesitancy about trying something new.

> **Familiar, yet fabulous:** It's important to know who you're cooking for and the kinds of foods they typically enjoy. Once you have this as your starting point, you can easily "veganize" these familiar favorites by eliminating the animal products and substituting vegan versions, such as vegan cheese on pizza and in lasagna, non-dairy milk in cream sauces and pudding, TVP and vegan beef crumbles in chili and tacos, and tempeh instead of tuna salad. For those who are more adventurous, try experimenting further by utilizing a similar flavor palette to create raw vegan dishes, such as spiraled zucchini "zoodles" with raw puttanesca and cashew parmesan or taco sliders with endive leaves stuffed with seasoned nut meat, cashew sour cream, and pico de gallo. Your guests will be so amazed at the versatility of plant-based foods they won't feel deprived.

> **Color, taste, and texture:** When creating a meal, think about how it will look on your plate. Food that is balanced is appealing to the eye and palate and is satisfying to eat. Envision the Color Wheel and complementary colors that work well when

paired together. You want vibrant, contrasting colors such as red and green, like tomatoes tossed with kale in a Mediterranean Quinoa Salad, or the bright pop of Roasted Red Pepper Harissa to dress up Baked Stuffed Zucchini Romesco. Think of Italian and Mexican food, with contrasting colors from roasted red and green peppers, fresh basil chiffonade over marinara, salsa and guacamole, or silvers of bright green scallion sprinkled over a mole sauce. Warm hued vegetables like carrot, butternut squash, or garnet yam intensify a plate and stimulate the appetite. Fresh chopped parsley scattered for garnish creates visual interest in an otherwise ordinary dish. Every meal you create should also strive for balance of the four tastes: salty, sweet, sour, and bitter, plus the occasional kick of spice, as well as umami for that savory quality many non-vegans crave. Think about the flavor profile you are creating every time you put together a meal. If it seems like "something's missing," consult your taste palate. Often a squeeze of lemon is all that's needed to perk up a dish. A variety of textures also adds a little intrigue to the meal. Including an array of crispy, crunchy, chewy, hard, soft, smooth, creamy, and silky textures in your meals gives your mouth a workout and stimulates your senses, which makes food more interesting and ultimately more satisfying.

Plating techniques: Think of your plate as an empty canvas, or a room that needs a feng shui makeover. You want to arrange items on your plate to establish a flow of energy that invites investigation and inspires contemplation with each forkful. A quick lesson in visual balance is to "think in threes," or odd numbers, which creates harmony. If there are two items on a plate, such as a portobello mushroom and baked potato plopped side by side, they will be competing for your attention and neither will win. Instead, choose three items and arrange them in a triangle, for example, mashed root vegetables such as garnet yam in a mound placed off center, steamed asparagus laid in a diagonal across the center of the plate, and roasted portobello placed at a 45 degree angle against the mashed yams. A simple garnish such as Tahini Dijon Dressing drizzled inside the circumference of the plate plus a sprinkle of thinly sliced green onion over the top will enhance the visual appeal.

Sauces, garnishes, and flavor bursts: Taking simple meals and adding layers of interest makes food exciting. Think of your entree as the main component in the center of the plate, then add a sauce on the bottom and a garnish on top to create the layers. A sauce finishes off a dish and pulls separate components together, as with the previously discussed portobello mushroom meal. It is often composed of a bright, pungent flavor, such as Dijon mustard or lemon and capers, that enhances a dish. Being heavy-handed on the seasonings could be overpowering (or as we foodies say, "too assertive"), but just enough can intrigue the senses. Garnishes add an element of color, texture, or both, and they likewise make an otherwise ordinary dish fabulous. Try garnishing a silky vegetable bisque soup with toasted pepitas, pair a wedge of Dirty Blondie Tart with a smooth, spicy maple pumpkin sauce topped with toasted coconut, or drizzle a creamy remoulade on top of crispy vegan crab cakes. If you really want to add the "wow factor" to your meals, experiment with "flavor bursts" composed of the four tastes taken to the extreme. I learned this technique from Chef Ken Bergeron, author of Vegetarian Cooking for Professionals and former executive chef and owner of It's Only Natural vegan restaurant in Middletown, CT. He once made me a simple lunch of Indonesian noodles a flavor adventure by topping the dish with a tablespoon of toasted coconut, toasted chopped peanuts, spicy red chili pepper flakes, lime zest and salt. These were all elements of the dish in concentrated form sprinkled over the top, which made twirling the noodles into this burst of flavor an adventure with each bite.

Ultimately, if it doesn't taste good, it will be tough to win people over. But the first step is to respect our heritage and learn to utilize the culturally appropriate spices and seasonings that make food taste delicious. Familiar foods, often aptly referred to as "comfort foods," represent an affiliation with a culture and are usually introduced during childhood where they are associated with security and happy memories. As members of a social group, many of us come to associate these food choices with our personal identity, and making the shift to veganism can be problematic if it's too dramatic a change. "An essential symbolic function of food is cultural identity. What one eats defines who one is, culturally speaking, and, conversely, who one is not."[2] Most of us enter into veganism with baggage and biases from our non-vegan family traditions and social customs. We assimilate into the environment in which we were raised with little thought about what we put into our mouths until we're exposed to alternatives. We're raised to believe that harming animals is

2. Kittler, P. G., Sucher, K. P., & Nahikian-Nelms, M. (2011). *Food and Culture*. USA: Wadsworth

wrong, and in the moment we realize that the food on our plate was once a living, joyful being, we recoil with horror, severing our cultural identity. Some of us may make these connections on our own with little influence from outside sources and immediately change our behaviors. But for most of us, it takes time to reflect on our habits and reconcile our behaviors with our beliefs. Be aware that these embedded culinary practices can be hurdles for many people to overcome when they are experiencing vegan versions of their favorite foods.

I once catered a bridal shower cooking party for 20 Italian women from Long Island where only the future bride was vegan. She boldly requested a traditional Italian themed menu and a main course of lasagna with summer vegetables. When one of the aunts came into the kitchen to look over the recipes and ingredients, she said not too quietly under her breath, "Tofu should never be allowed anywhere near lasagna." I reassured her that the flavors of the sauce and vegan ricotta I was making would be so delicious and familiar that she'd never even notice she was eating tofu. She smirked and uttered, "We'll see," as she walked away. Later in the afternoon, I pulled the bubbly tray of lasagna out of the oven and served everyone their gooey, luscious portions topped with a sprinkle of cashew parmesan and basil chiffonade. I heard nothing but raves, and even better, the skeptical aunt walked over to the tray and cut herself a second generous portion while remarking, "OK, you were right. I'm surprised it's so good. Shocked even." I thanked her for being open-minded and was glad she enjoyed it.

Cooking with Confidence and Conviction

When I speak with vegan friends who complain about the lack of enthusiasm of non-vegan friends and family members to try their food, I always ask, "How did you pitch it?" They explain that they usually bring a vegan dish to a get-together which they quietly eat alone, shuddering in revulsion as everyone around them devours various animal body parts. Or they complain, "Nobody wanted to touch what I brought because it's vegan." Sound familiar? While I can completely understand the frustration, we have to remember that not everyone is as enlightened as we are. It's our job to be positive and non-judgmental, despite the recognition that others may still be so fully entrenched in their upbringing and societal norms that they can't imagine exploring beyond their safe boundaries.

I could very easily have become upset when I was chided for making lasagna with tofu, but I recognized that this comment was made from an uninformed perspective, by a woman whose rigid adherence to traditions prevented her from even considering there was any other way to make Italian food than what she knew. As a vegan activist, it's my role to convince people otherwise, or at least to open their eyes to the possibility. I do this by speaking with confidence and conviction, not sarcasm or condescension. I know my food is amazing and I don't need to convince anyone of that. But what I do need to do is convince them to *trust* me. That's the difference. And that's what I mean by how you pitch it. This is not about being disingenuous like a salesman who's trying to unload a lemon. Rather, it's *trusting yourself* to be a spokesperson for the animals, standing by your beliefs, being unapologetic for your passion, and knowing that you are doing what's ethically right. Tell them how much they're going to love the food you brought. Cut them a serving and put it on their plate. Ask them to just give it a try, and reassure them they'll be amazed. Be careful, however. It's not about being arrogant, egotistical, or superior, which will only shun those who are not yet receptive to your message. Rather, it's striking the inviting tone of friendly vanguard by staying positive, poised, and passionate in your vegan convictions. That authenticity demonstrates an integrity that's compelling to even the most critical skeptics.

Picky Eaters

I've cooked for many self-described "picky eaters" in my years as a vegan chef, and the one thing I've discovered they all have in common is anxiety about the unknown. Somewhere, at some point in their life, they made an unpleasant association with a certain food — whether it was the taste, the texture, how it looked on their plate, or just some random irrational disdain for an otherwise innocent fruit or vegetable — and that association stuck with them. Shunning the forbidden food gives them a sense of control, the safety part of the Omnivore's Paradox. It enables them to push aside all those uncomfortable feelings worrying about trying something new and different so they can get on with the task of eating. To them, consuming food is more a chore than a pleasure; it's something they have to do to physically exist. The fewer the surprises, the more tolerable the process. While this coping mechanism may have served to minimize their anxieties in the past, it has left them with a limited palate and a rigid unwillingness to experiment with new foods, especially vegan ones. It can be a tough challenge to win over this type of eater. What has worked for the picky eaters I've coached is a three step process:

> *Set ground rules.* Have them agree to give the new food a try. Thank them for their willingness. Refrain from making judgments.

> *Create a safe space.* Let them know it's ok if they don't like it. They won't offend anyone if they spit it out.

> *Engage their curiosity.* Ask them to describe foods they enjoy while they're eating something new. Demonstrate how fun and delicious food can be. This is the adventurous side of the Omnivore's Paradox.

I once taught a cooking class where the food sample I had prepared was an olive tapenade "vegan caviar" on crostini. I noticed one student was sitting in her chair not eating, so I asked if she had gotten her hor d'oeuvres. She shook her head, crinkled her nose, and said, "No, I don't like olives." I told her she would absolutely not offend me if she tried it and spit it into her napkin because it repulsed her, but that she was here in this class to learn and owed it to herself to give it a taste. So she hesitatingly took a slice from me and walked away while I went back to serving others. A few minutes later she walked up to my table with a strange look on her face. "You spit it out, didn't you?" I teased. "That's ok if you did. I'm just glad you tried it!" She responded with a tentative smile, "Actually, I came up for seconds. It was delicious." And of course I loaded that second helping of crusty bread with a good slathering of tapenade for her to enjoy. It's the kind of response I always love getting.

Pleasing Kids

Never underestimate the potential of just being a positive vegan role model to influence people, especially kids. Tap into their natural curiosity about life and encourage their creativity. Kids are continually shaping their identities through their daily activities and you have the potential to influence their adventurous spirit with food. Make it fun. Encourage them to experiment. Teach them lessons. Let them get messy. Roll up their sleeves and give them a job. When I was a little girl, my mom had me cut up all the vegetables for dinner when I got home from school. She showed me how to use a vegetable peeler and a knife and told me to "cut them uniformly." I learned that by cutting the vegetables the same size they would cook evenly. I learned math when she told me to "cut the potatoes into quarters." She showed me how to set the timer and explained that cooking time varied depending on the food. She let me decorate my salad with carrot ribbons and sliced cucumber I had scored with a fork to make it look like zebra stripes. All of these little tasks gave me a sense of confidence in the kitchen, and cooking became a fun experience I looked forward to, with the meal at the end the reward.

Nearly half of my clients come to me for cooking lessons because a son or daughter has told them they want to go vegan. I think it's so great not only that children today have connected their heart and head — they love animals and realize they have a choice to not eat them — and that their parents are supportive of this choice. This is tremendous progress both with education and personal liberty. I often encourage parents to empower their children to make healthy food choices by letting them help create the dinner menu. Start by having them write a list of fruits, vegetables, beans, and other foods they enjoy eating. Then go to an online vegan recipe resource like www.VegWeb.com where you can enter a vegetable in the search box and find dozens of recipes made with it. Pick a healthy recipe that you can make together and have the kids help with finding the ingredients at the grocery store. The hands-on involvement of finding the ingredients and preparing them at home will take the mystery out of the food and add to the sense of accomplishment and enjoyment when eating it.

Another fun activity is a healthy scavenger hunt. Give kids a shopping list of pantry staples and ask them to help find them at the grocery store. Stick to items found in the produce aisle, canned goods, and bulk bins. Avoid going down aisles with processed foods loaded with salt, sugar, and fat. Encourage them to read labels and understand what the ingredients mean. Age-appropriate lessons like these can help develop healthy eating habits that will last a lifetime.

Children also have a desire to do good in the world. Remind them that eating vegan helps the planet and reduces animal suffering. Choose products with minimal packaging and explain the importance of recycling. Use cloth shopping bags from home and only buy what you will use. Let them know that their actions are helping feed people around the world and preserving the planet for future generations.

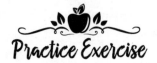

Practice Exercise

This is the time to put your skills into practice. Experiment first with your own meals by making them visually appealing using some of the plating techniques discussed in this chapter. Take a look at my Instagram feed @wellonwheels for some inspiring photos of recipes found in this book. Once you're feeling confident with a few dishes that will impress your guests, consider hosting a dinner party (or at least invite a good friend to a home-cooked meal). Here are some tips to help make your dinner a success:

Plan Ahead. Find out what foods and flavors your guests enjoy. Stick with familiar favorites that can easily be veganized. (See Chapter 9 for recipe ideas.)

Create a Menu. Whether it's a casual dinner for two, a summer picnic, or a gourmet feast, you'll want to write out your list of dishes and decide how they will be served.

Set the Table. This time you want to do it literally as well as figuratively. A pretty table that includes a vase of fresh flowers, a clean tablecloth, and a tidy arrangement of plates and silverware is inviting. Your enthusiasm will also set the tone.

Plate It Up. Get a squeeze bottle and have fun with sauces. Chop up some fresh herbs and use edible flowers for garnish. Make it pretty. Prepare for the Wow Factor.

Have Fun. Envision your guests joyfully sipping cocktails and raving about the amazing food you've prepared for them. Make this an experience to remember, and it will be.

Chapter 8

The Vegan Kitchen

Let's assume you've established a 100% Vegan Kitchen in your household. There will be no divided pantries, no separate refrigerator space relegated to meat, eggs, and cheese, no hidden stashes of Milk Duds and Cheetos, nothing to sabotage your efforts to maintain a vegan lifestyle for yourself and those you love. Nope. You're starting with a clean slate and you need to establish a strong foundation upon which to build. This can feel overwhelming at first, but as you set your mind to it and follow the tips outlined in this chapter, you will create a sanctuary that emanates these values.

You don't need the most expensive, top of the line products to make exquisite food, but with regards to ingredients and equipment, you often get what you pay for. That said, I will make recommendations for various budgets as well as offer my personal preferences as suggestions. This is what I've come to favor over the years, but that doesn't necessarily mean that other products aren't equally good. It also doesn't mean you need to splurge on everything all at once and go broke in the process. Buy what you're comfortable with when starting out, upgrade when necessary, and consider every purchase an investment that will make cooking a joy.

Kitchen Equipment

It's important to equip your kitchen with the right tools of the trade so that you'll not only be safe and feel comfortable, but also so that you and your family will come to enjoy the cooking process itself and not see it as an obstacle to being vegan. When I first started out in my own kitchen prior to becoming a personal chef, I didn't even have a cutting board. I used to hold an apple in the palm of my left hand and pray that the serrated steak knife I was gingerly holding in my right hand wouldn't slip. Yes, it was bad. But if I can get over the hurdle, so can you.

APPLIANCES

Take care of the major investments by equipping your kitchen with the right appliances based on your budget. If the price tags seem unaffordable at first, you can often find kitchen appliances at thrift stores or on Craigslist at a bargain. I managed with a hand-me-down blender and $29.99 Black & Decker food processor for years before I became fully committed to vegan cooking. Once I invested in some higher quality appliances, it became much easier and more enjoyable to experiment with new recipes.

> **Food processor:** Get the biggest you can afford (I recommend 14-cup) as this will save time when making large batches of mixtures such as pate, nut crusts, vegan cheeses, and bean dips. Cuisinart is a reliable standard.

High speed blender: I use mine nearly every day for smoothies, sauces, and nut milks. You can get by with something basic like a Waring, and even a Ninja or NutriBullet will get the job done, but when you're feeling confident and ready to splurge, go with a Vitamix or Blendtec. You can save a little money by buying one reconditioned directly from the manufacturer's website.

Immersion blender: For pureeing hot soups to a smooth consistency, this is indispensable. If you get one with a bowl attachment, you can also use it for processing smaller jobs. This is great for making a whipped "cream" or single serving of sauce. I take it with me wherever I cook because it's much easier to transport than my blender and food processor! An immersion blender with attachments is also a decent, affordable option before you're ready to purchase two separate appliances. Cuisinart and Braun are some good manufacturers.

TOOLS

These essential tools will make cooking easy and fun, and you'll feel like a pro when you use them.

- » knives – 8" chef's knife, serrated knife, paring knife (Wustof and Global are good, affordable brands)
- » knife sharpener and honing steel
- » skillet – 10" stainless steel, 10" enameled non-stick, 10" cast iron (look for The Lodge brand)
- » pots – Dutch oven (6 qt), 5–6 qt. pasta pot, 1–2 qt. sauce pot with lids. I like Le Creuset's gorgeous enameled pots which are perfect for chili and

soup; All-Clad is the best when it comes to every-day cookware, but if you can't afford that, choose heavy stainless steel Calphalon or Cuisinart.

» metal colander and fine mesh sieve
» mixing bowls, measuring cups (wet and dry) and measuring spoons
» wooden cutting board (avoid plastic or ceramic which rapidly dull your knife)

GADGETS

I'm not a fan of gadgets that serve just one purpose because they just clutter storage space, but these essentials make kitchen chores a breeze. Except where noted, I really like OXO brand for most of these.

» garlic press (Zyliss is the best)
» metal tongs
» metal and plastic spatulas
» wooden spoons of different sizes
» ladle
» vegetable peeler and zester
» box grater
» mandolin slicer
» saladacco spiral slicer "spiralizer"

Pantry Staples

The key to staying vegan in the home is to stock your pantry with staples that are versatile, healthful, and have a long shelf life so you'll be ready for any kitchen emergency. After a long day at work, the last thing you'll want to do is go grocery shopping with all the other weary shoppers searching for that one item you don't have on hand. Keep a list on your refrigerator of items that are running low and stock up when you have the time to shop.

» bulk grains (brown rice, millet, wild rice, amaranth, teff, corn meal)
» bulk nuts and seeds (almonds, walnuts, pecans, pistachios, pine nuts, quinoa, chia seeds, flax seeds, hemp seeds, pumpkin seeds, sesame seeds, sunflower seeds)
» bulk dry legumes (black-eyed peas, brown lentil, French lentil, red lentil)
» pasta (Italian style, rice pasta, Asian rice noodles, soba noodles)
» canned tomatoes (Muir Glen fire-roasted are fabulous!), beans (black, butter, kidney, cannelini, pinto, garbanzo), coconut milk, jackfruit
» non-dairy milks (rice, almond, hemp, coconut, soy, flax, cashew - pick your favorite!)
» sea vegetables (nori sheets, dulse flakes, arame)
» oils (olive, toasted sesame, canola, unrefined coconut, Earth Balance margarine)
» condiments (balsamic vinegar, apple cider vinegar, Dijon mustard, yellow mustard, spicy brown mustard, horseradish, hot sauce, tamari, pickles, nut butters, tahini, jam, etc.)
» bulk herbs and spices (basil, oregano, rosemary, cumin, chili powder, coriander, turmeric, curry powder, garlic powder, onion powder, nutritional yeast)
» baking products (flour, corn starch, baking soda, baking powder, cocoa powder, vanilla extract)
» sweeteners (agave syrup, rice syrup, maple syrup, evaporated cane sugar, brown sugar, Stevia)

Personally, I recommend holding off on stocking your pantry with dessert ingredients such as flours, sweeteners, and chocolate, partly because they're expensive, but mostly because I believe desserts should be kept to a minimum to stay healthy and balanced. However, for holidays, special occasions, and opportunities to win over skeptical non-vegans, an occasional sweet treat can be essential.

This is where I began nearly twenty years ago. You will learn what your favorites are the more you experiment. While I didn't include items like vegan cheeses, plant-based meats, and other quick fix convenience foods on this list, I do understand they can be essential "transition foods" to help wean non-vegans off animal products, so I will offer a list of recommended substitutions next.

Substitutions

At first, the prospect of switching to a vegan diet can feel daunting for non-vegans because they may feel as if they're giving up more than they're gaining. However, when you remind them that the foods they are no longer consuming generally are not needed for optimal health and can also promote disease with their added saturated fat and cholesterol, their acidifying and inflammatory effects on the body, and if non-organic, their residual hormones, antibiotics and other pharmaceuticals, they will understand why they really don't want to be eating them. What they're gaining in this process is not only physical health, but peace of mind, clarity of conscience, freedom from exploitation, and a deeper emotional connection to the animals. This is worth far more than the temporary pleasure of one's palate when ingesting a plateful of suffering. Besides, vegan versions of traditional favorites taste just as good as, if not better than, the original.

The following list serves as basic guidelines to help you with meal planning for breakfast, lunch and dinner, as well as the occasional baked goods and snacks. Rest assured concerned family and friends, we've got you covered.

MEAT

Tofu: This versatile fermented soybean based product comes in two styles, Chinese and Japanese. The Chinese style is a firmer, "meatier" texture which works well in stir-fry recipes, baked cutlets and scrambles. Its flavor can be enhanced by sitting in flavorful marinades. The Japanese style is smoother and silkier and is often cubed in miso soup. It can also be blended into smoothies and puddings for an extra boost of protein.

Tempeh: Another fermented soy product, tempeh has a denser texture than tofu and is also higher in protein content. It can be simply pan-fried in oil with salt and pepper or baked with a sauce. Be careful when using a marinade since tempeh will soak it up like a sponge.

Seitan: Made from wheat gluten, the protein of wheat flour, seitan is a high protein meat substitute. It is typically seasoned with soy sauce, garlic and ginger and used in stir-frys and sautés. It can also be sliced and breaded like a meat cutlet.

Beans and Legumes: There is a vast array of options here, whether using them in a soup, mixed with a marinara to make a Bolognese sauce, blended into a dip or sandwich spread, or mixed into a salad. They're high in fiber and low in calories, so they'll fill you up without fattening you up.

Textured Vegetable Protein (TVP): This dried protein mixture can be hydrated with water and added to chili, sauce or soup to elicit a "ground beef" texture. It's also a great addition to a vegan pot pie filling.

Faux Meat: There are so many meat alternatives on the market that provide taste and texture that are so close to the real thing that some people have trouble telling the difference. Whether they're chicken strips, nuggets, sausage, burgers or bacon, clever manufacturers have come up with vegan alternatives for nearly all of these favorites to help wean meat eaters from the animal addiction. See the Appendix for a list of products.

DAIRY

Milk: Rice milk has a naturally sweet flavor and can be found in blends with carob, chocolate and even Rice Nog for the holidays. Oat milk is another grain based dairy alternative. Almond is the most common of the nut milks, but coconut milk and cashew milk are also becoming widely available. Hemp milk is quickly gaining popularity as a dairy alternative because it's a complete protein and high in Omega-3 oil. Quinoa, chia, sunflower and flax seed milks are also available. Soy milk has long been a staple for vegans and it's also popular as a non-dairy creamer for coffee. You can also make your own nut milk by blending one cup of nuts (soaked in water at least an hour, drained and rinsed) with 4 cups of fresh water, a drizzle of agave syrup and a pinch of sea salt. Strain through a cheesecloth if desired.

Yogurt and Sour Cream: You can easily find soy and coconut based nondairy cultured yogurts and smooth and creamy sour cream that are similar in flavor and texture to the traditional dairy versions. These work great in dips or in baked goods.

Cheese and Cream Cheese: There used to be a time when the only vegan cheese you could find were blocks of flavorless processed foods that were about as appetizing as sliced wax. We are fortunate today to have nondairy cheeses that melt, stretch, spread and taste so authentic that you won't even miss that other stuff. Try some nut-based varieties of fermented cheese spread on a cracker or crumbled in a salad.

Ice Cream: There are just as many options here as there are milk alternatives, and you can find flavor combinations that are decadent on a sultry summer afternoon. Ben & Jerry's has even gotten into nondairy ice cream production after years of demand from eager customers.

Butter: While margarine has long been a butter substitute, it can also be loaded with hydrogenated oil and trans fats which are not good for you. Plus, some margarines include whey or casein from dairy among their ingredients, so be sure to read labels. Earth Balance is a blessing to vegans.

EGGS

Commercial Egg Replacers: Follow Your Heart "Vegan Egg," The Vegg, Beyond Eggs, and EnerG are commercial egg replacers that can be substituted in any baking recipe. They can also be used to make your favorite scramble, frittata or even a crepe. Who knew you could eat like a Parisian aristocrat and still be cruelty free!

DIY Egg Replacers: Ground flax seed is an easy substitute for eggs in baking. When mixed with water, it gets a gelatinous consistency that works well as a binder, plus you get the added benefit of extra fiber and Omega-3 oil. 1 tbsp ground flax seed plus 3 tbsp of water = 1 egg. Other substitutes that are the equivalent of one egg and can be used in baking include ¼ cup mashed banana, ¼ cup applesauce, or ¼ cup blended silken tofu. If you just need a leavening agent (something to make your baked goods rise), try using 1 tsp vinegar plus 1 tbsp baking soda for one egg.

Mayo: Traditional mayonnaise is made with eggs and oil. There are several commercial vegan mayonnaise brands on the market that look just like real mayo and taste fabulous spread on a sandwich or blended into salads. Some favorites are Just Mayo, Earth Balance Mindful Mayo, and Veganaise. You can also make your own vegan mayo by pureeing ¼ cup silken tofu with 1 tsp apple cider vinegar, 1 tsp lemon juice, 1 tsp Dijon mustard and a little salt. Alternatively, you can blend ½ cup raw cashews with ¼ water in place of the tofu for a raw cashew mayo.

WHAT ABOUT GLUTEN?

Although some people avoid eating gluten (the protein found in wheat, barley and rye), it is technically vegan and ok to eat if you are not sensitive to it. However, many vegan products on the market today contain highly refined wheat gluten which one should be careful about eating in large quantities because wheat is acidifying to the body and can cause inflammation, which can create imbalance and lead to a host of health problems[1]. In addition, wheat is mucus forming and can cause sinus congestion, headaches, and cold-like flu symptoms.[2] For these reasons, recipes in this cookbook contain gluten-free recommendations where needed to accommodate those with celiac disease, gluten sensitivities, and wheat allergies. Gluten-free flours made from garbanzo beans, fava beans, potato starch, sorghum, coconut, and brown rice are substituted for wheat flour and combined with either xanthan gum, tapioca starch, or corn starch to take the place of gluten and prevent the baked goods from being too crumbly.

WHAT ABOUT OIL, SUGAR, AND SALT?

Some people follow a whole foods, plant-based diet for health reasons, and they avoid all forms of added fat, refined sugar, and salt. If you have a history of heart disease and diabetes, you may want to consider going this route. Cleveland Clinic Cardiologist Dr. Caldwell Esselstyn and Cornell University Professor Emeritus of Nutritional Biochemistry Dr. T. Colin Campbell have done extensive research on the connection between diet and cardiovascular health and are pioneers in the growing field of plant-based preventive medicine. Their studies have shown that a diet high in whole foods like fruits, vegetables, beans, and grains can prevent and even reverse common degenerative diseases such as cardiovascular disease and Type II diabetes. There are many excellent resources available that can provide guidance for maintaining this lifestyle. A good place to start are the documentaries *Forks Over Knives* and *Plant Pure Nation*, as well as the websites by the same name.

---

1. Karin de Punder, and Leo Pruimboom. *"The Dietary Intake of Wheat and Other Cereal Grains and Their Role in Inflammation."* Nutrients, vol. 5, no. 3, 2013, pp. 771–787.
2. *"Favorite Holiday Foods Making You Sick?; Gluten Could Be Culprit, Says Nationally Recognized Expert Carol Fenster, Ph.D."* PR Newswire, 2006, p. n/a.

Sample Meal Plan

Substituting a veggie burger for a hamburger or almond milk for cow's milk is pretty straightforward, but sometimes it helps to have an idea of what to prepare on a daily basis for breakfast, lunch, and dinner. This alleviates any sense of disorientation a non-vegan might feel when suddenly immersed in a vegan household. What follows is a seven-day meal plan that incorporates the basic principles of a whole foods plant based diet while balancing protein, carbohydrate, fat, vitamins, and minerals (based on nutrition recommendations by Nancy Berkoff, RD of the nonprofit Vegetarian Resource Group[3]).

Please note that this is NOT MEDICAL ADVICE. Everyone has his or her own individual energy and dietary needs, so be sure to consult your health care professional to determine whether these suggestions will work for you and your family members. The purpose of this list is to demonstrate the wide variety of foods available that can be eaten on a daily basis. Recipes can be found in the following chapter.

BREAKFAST IDEAS

- » 2 melon slices, 2 pancakes with ¼ cup chopped pecans, cinnamon, and diced apple
- » smoothie made with 1 banana, ½ cup berries, 1 kale leaf and 1 cup non-dairy milk
- » ¾ cup cooked oatmeal with ½ cup dried figs, 6 walnuts, 1 tbsp flax/chia/hemp seeds, 1 cup non-dairy milk
- » 1 orange, cranberry streusel muffin with 2 tbsp nut butter
- » 1 cup puffed millet cereal, topped with ¼ cup raspberries, ¼ cup raisins, ¼ cup slivered al-

---

3. *"Vegan Menu for People with Diabetes,"* by Nancy Bekoff, RD, https://www.vrg.org/journal/vj2003issue2/2003_issue2_diabetes.php

monds, 1 tbsp flax/chia/hemp seeds, ¼ tsp cinnamon, 8 oz. enriched non-dairy milk
» tostadas: brown rice tortilla with ¼ cup un-fried beans, 2 tablespoons vegan cheese, ½ cup vegan beef crumbles sautéed with chopped onions and peppers, 1 teaspoon cumin, ½ cup salsa
» southwestern tofu scramble with peppers, onions and mushrooms and ½ cup salsa

LUNCH IDEAS

» 1 cup rootsy chowder with 4 oz. buffalo tofu and 1 cup sesame green beans
» 6-inch pita stuffed with 2 oz. hummus, lettuce, tomatoes, and cucumbers, 1 cup shredded cabbage with 1-½ tbsp vegan mayonnaise
» Romaine lettuce salad with 1 tbsp dried berries, ¼ cup slivered almonds, 1 tbsp flax/chia/hemp seeds, and fat-free salad dressing
» Tempeh Tartar on Avocado Toast with clementine wedges
» 2 veggie burgers on shredded head of lettuce, sliced tomato, and shredded carrots and sliced cucumber, ½ avocado, ¼ cup salsa
» 1 cup eggless egg salad on endive leaves
» 1 cup Berbere Spiced Lentil Soup with sautéed kale and ½ cup brown rice

SNACK IDEAS

» ½ cup fresh grapes (or frozen in the summer), 6 walnuts
» 2 cups air popped popcorn with 2 teaspoons nutritional yeast and a pinch of sea salt

- » 1 orange, pear, apple, grapefruit, peach, or whatever fruit is in season
- » 2 tbsp peanut butter on sliced apple
- » ½ cup baked veggie chips with ½ cup salsa
- » 4 dried figs, 6 pecans
- » 1 cup vanilla non-dairy milk soaked with 2 tbsp chia seeds until pudding-like, 1 sliced banana, 2 tbsp pistachios or slivered almonds

DINNER IDEAS

- » 1 cup chili over ½ cup rice, ½ cup steamed greens
- » Baked eggplant (½ cup), ½ cup tomato sauce, oregano, ½ cup cannelini beans, ⅓ cup quinoa
- » ½ cup steamed broccoli with 1/4 cup red peppers, 1 steamed, baked, or roasted sweet potato with ½ teaspoon curry powder and 2 tbsp vegan sour cream
- » 6 oz. grilled portobello steak, 1 cup mashed root veggies and braised Swiss chard
- » 4 oz. barbecue jackfruit with ½ cup world peas salad
- » 4 oz. pan-fried tempeh with Dijon agave glaze, ½ cup sauteed kale and onions, ½ cup brown rice
- » 4 oz. pecan crusted tempeh, 1 cup mashed root vegetables with steamed asparagus

Special Menus

Although the above meals can be eaten on a daily basis, they can also become menus for special occasions with a few simple embellishments so you can "dress for success." Start with a humble dish like Mediterranean Quinoa Salad pressed into a 1 cup measuring cup then inverted onto a plate and surrounded by a colorful sauce like Parsley Pistou and topped with a sprinkle of toasted pine nuts. For dessert, take a Chocolate Kahlua Brownie and drizzle with chocolate ganache, then top with a big dollop of Coconut Whip and garnish with toasted coconut flakes. The components are elevated to create a gourmet presentation, with very little effort. This is how you transform everyday recipes into vegan feasts for the senses. Here are some ideas to get you started impressing non-vegan family and friends.

Valentine's Day: Some thoughts that immediately come to mind for this holiday are red foods, chocolate, and aphrodisiacs such as avocado, asparagus, spices, and dates. The meal I would create would be built around simple recipes dressed up for the occasion. Menu: Tempeh Tartare on Avocado Toast Points with edible flower garnish; Baked Stuffed Filet of Tofu on a bed of sautéed kale and Garnet Yam Hash; Chocolate Kahlua Brownies with Chocolate Ganache and Fresh Berries, plus a sprinkle of cinnamon and cocoa powder to decorate the plate.

St. Patrick's Day: Green is the theme for this holiday. Start with a Garden Veggie Soup topped with a drizzle of Parsley Pistou. For the entree, serve a hearty Tempeh Stroganoff with Broccoli on top of mashed potatoes.

Vernal Equinox: This is the time of year to be thinking about a cleanse. Focus on light, raw foods that are in season. Menu: Shaved Brussels Sprout Salad; Seared Mushroom "Scallops" with Lemon Caper Sauce on Sautéed Spinach and Linguini.

Summer Picnic in the Raw: This is my favorite time of year, and I let the garden dictate the menu. When summer vegetables like zucchini are in abundance, it's time to get out the spiralizer. Menu: World Peas Salad; Zucchini Ribbons with Cashew Cheese Sauce and Sun-dried Tomato Marinara; Strawberry Shortcake with Coconut Whip Cream.

ThanksLiving: For a stress-free holiday, I often take a shortcut and make a prepared holiday roast from Tofurky, Field Roast or Gardein then augment with my favorite sides. If you want to do it all from scratch, my Pecan Crusted Tempeh makes a good centerpiece on top of Mashed Root Veggies, Brussels Sprouts Amandine, Roasted Asparagus, all slathered with Crimini Mushroom Gravy. My Pumpkin Streusel Tart is the perfect way to end the meal.

Holiday Time: If you're planning a party for the winter holidays, think of finger food as well as entrees that can be made in large portions and served on pretty platters. This will minimize the work involved with preparing food for the masses. Also consider components of your meal that can be utilized in a variety of ways. For example, Olive Tapenade can be spread on crostini, stirred into a dip with pureed cannelini beans for crudites, used as a filling with roasted veggies in wraps, and tossed with pasta, beans, cherry tomatoes, and baby spinach for a simple main dish.

New Year's Brunch: I like to start the new year by indulging in warming comfort food. To me, this is the perfect way to cozy up with friends and family and relax after a night of partying. These are easy do-ahead recipes that can be eaten warm or cold, so you don't need much effort in the morning. Menu: Apple Bread Pudding with Maple Pecan Praline and Coconut Whip; Tofu Florentine Quiche; Home-fried Smoked Paprika Potatoes with Sriracha; Cranberry Streusel Muffins.

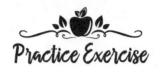

Practice Exercise

You now have a foundation for a vegan kitchen and the skills for inspiring others to adopt a vegan lifestyle. Start with positive thoughts for the future as you fully embrace all of the concepts discussed in these chapters.

> » **Envision the life you want to live, and live it.**
> » **Surround yourself with those who support your vision and encourage you rather than bring you down.**
> » **Challenge yourself to move into your discomfort zone.**
> » **Have compassion for yourself and extend that compassion to others.**
> » **Honor and respect your true nature.**
> » **Be a beacon of light guiding others on the vegan journey.**

Life's greatest challenges can push you to your limits (and beyond!), leading you to grow in ways you never imagined possible. Embrace those challenges as a gift from the universe, and know that every difficulty you encounter is an opportunity to learn more about yourself and others so that you can become a better activist for the animals.

Part 2

Compassionate Cuisine

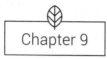

Chapter 9

Recipes

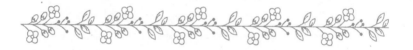

What follows is a collection of some of my favorite recipes I've used to entice family, friends, co-workers, students, and clients into embracing a vegan lifestyle. For photo inspiration, follow my Instagram feed (@wellonwheels) and use the hashtag #EZPZVegan. I use the techniques described in the previous chapters to set the foundation, then I win them over with fabulous flavors and beautiful presentations. Let me emphasize that it's critical to do both. I once had a client come to me requesting the perfect recipe that would win over her reluctant boyfriend and "make him go vegan." While I'd like to think there are magical recipes that can achieve this lofty goal, the truth is we can't make anyone change if they're not ready to. This is why it's so important to engage in the kinds of conversations presented in this book on a regular basis. My advice to her was to guide her boyfriend through the process by piquing his curiosity, inspiring his empathy, and encouraging his adventurous spirit such that eating vegan with her would eventually become the new norm. And whenever you cook, make compassion the main course. That said, I hope these recipes make that transition easy and enjoyable! Below are some tips to always keep in mind when preparing food to make it appealing for your guests so that they'll want to dig right in.

Guidelines for Plating

Keep food off the rim of the plate: Think of the plate as a picture frame with an appropriate portion of food arranged inside the borders.

Strive for balance of colors: Contrasting colors like bright red and green "pop" on the plate and are inviting to the eyes. Try to avoid a sea of beige which screams: *boring!*

Height makes food appealing and inviting: Arrange your food in layers on the plate with a sauce on the bottom, components placed beside each other, with an attractive garnish on top. Often just a little added height is enough to engage one's anticipation of the meal.

Cut ingredients neatly: Sharply sliced veggies, angle cut, or diced in uniform pieces will make a dish look crisp and professional. Avoid haphazardly cutting or sloppily arranging elements on the plate.

Keep it simple: A natural arrangement on the plate without an overabundance of elements presents a crisp design. Too elaborate or gimmicky can appear contrived, and a cluttered plate can look sloppy (unless it's a potluck where you're trying to cram as much as you can on your plate!). Also, avoid that single sprig of parsley for a garnish.

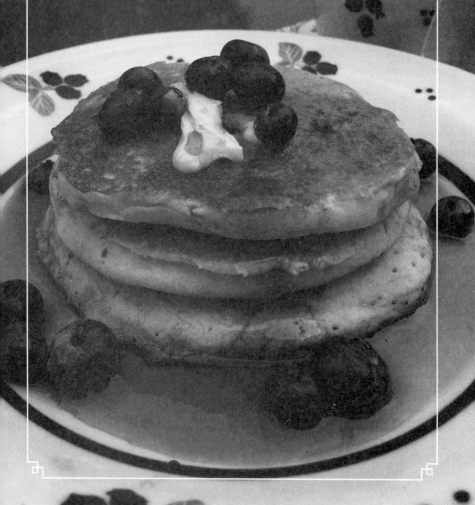

Breakfast

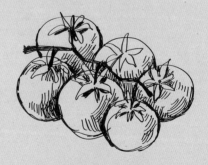

Breakfast

Start the morning off right with these fla-
vor-packed recipes. Some are savory, some
sweet, and some are a combination of both.
To make your mornings easier, consider recipes
that can be made ahead the night before for an
easy grab-and-go treat to take with you to the office. Others are meant for a lazy weekend morning,
perfect for treating your significant other. If you've
got a whole family to cook for, choose a variety of
foods that are packed with protein and accompany
them with fresh fruit, a glass of orange juice, and a
handful of nuts to munch on.

SOUTHWESTERN TOFU SCRAMBLE

(serves 2 to 4)

> *This colorful and flavorful recipe works well on a brunch buffet or hearty weekend breakfast. Serve with a side of Smoked Paprika Home-fried Potatoes.*

INGREDIENTS

» 2 tbsp olive oil
» 1 cup yellow onion, diced
» 1 clove garlic, crushed
» 1 cup red bell pepper, diced
» 1 cup green pepper, diced
» 4 oz. mushrooms, sliced
» 1 lb. extra firm tofu, patted dry and crumbled
» ½ tsp sea salt
» 1–2 tbsp nutritional yeast
» 1 tsp turmeric
» 1 tbsp Dijon mustard
» 1 tbsp tomato paste

Sauté the onion and garlic in the oil until onion softens. Add the red and green pepper and cook for 5 to 10 minutes, or until soft. Add the mushrooms and continue to sauté until they become soft. Add the crumbled tofu and sprinkle sea salt, nutritional yeast, and turmeric over it. Stir in remaining ingredients and mix well. Continue to cook until water evaporates and tofu is heated through.

BREAKFAST TOSTADAS

(serves 2)

> *This is a great recipe when you make a little extra tofu scramble and have leftovers the next day. Heap some on top of a tortilla along with a few tasty fixings and bake it in the oven for a satisfying morning meal.*

INGREDIENTS

- » 2 12 inch flour tortillas (gluten-free rice tortillas can be substituted)
- » ½ cup chipotle cashew aioli
- » 2 cups tofu scramble
- » 4 leaves of kale (lacinato or curly), stems removed
- » ½ cup salsa
- » 1 avocado, cut in half and each half thinly sliced into 8 pieces
- » ¼ cup sofritos

Preheat oven to 375°F. Place two tortillas on a baking sheet and spread a thin layer of chipotle cashew aioli over each. Top each with about a cup of tofu scramble. You can also substitute canned black beans, refried beans, or even hummus in place of the tofu scramble for variation. Remove stems from kale, stack leaves, then thinly slice into a chiffonade. Spread kale on top of the tofu scramble, then top with a scoop of salsa. Bake in the oven for 10 to 15 minutes, or until kale has wilted and tortilla is golden brown and beginning to crisp. Remove from oven and lay sliced avocado in a spiral pattern, then top with a couple spoonfuls of sofrito. You can also drizzle more chipotle cashew aioli from a squeeze bottle in a zig-zag over the top for an extra layer of flavor.

SMOKED PAPRIKA HOME-FRIED POTATOES

(serves 2 to 4)

> *Potatoes are one of my comfort foods, and this recipe is reminiscent of my post-college, pre-vegan days standing in line at the local greasy spoon, waiting for a pile of hot and spicy potatoes slathered in Cholula sauce to sooth my early morning hangover. This vegan version hits the spot (hangover and hot sauce optional).*

INGREDIENTS

» 4 medium sized red potatoes, cut into 1-inch chunks
» 1 tbsp olive oil
» 1 medium yellow onion, diced
» 2 tbsp vegan margarine
» 1 tsp sea salt
» 1 tsp smoked paprika
» ¼ tsp curry powder
» ¼ tsp cayenne pepper
» ¼ tsp fresh cracked black pepper

Bring a large pot of water to a boil. Add potatoes and cook until tender but still firm, about 5 to 10 minutes. Drain and let cool. Meanwhile, in a large skillet (cast iron works best), heat olive oil over medium high heat and add onion. Cook for about 5 minutes, stirring often, until soft and slightly browned. Add vegan margarine, potato cubes, salt, paprika, curry powder, cayenne and black pepper and stir to coat. Cook until potatoes are warmed through and slightly browned, about 10 minutes. Serve hot with a good douse of your favorite hot sauce (I like Cholula, Frank's, Sriracha, or Tabasco).

PERFECT PANCAKES

(makes 8 to 9 pancakes)

> *This is my Sunday morning treat, especially after shoveling snow or raking leaves.*

INGREDIENTS

» 1 cup all-purpose flour (or substitute 1 cup all-purpose gluten-free flour plus ½ tsp xanthan gum)
» 2 tsp baking powder
» ½ tsp sea salt
» ½ tsp cinnamon
» 1 cup unsweetened almond milk
» 2 tbsp agave syrup
» 1 tsp vanilla
» 1 tbsp coconut oil, melted
» ½ cup chopped pecans

Mix together all the dry ingredients in a large bowl. In a separate bowl, whisk together the almond milk, agave syrup, vanilla, and oil, then whisk into the dry ingredients. Stir well to combine, then add chopped pecans. You may need to add a few tbsp of water to achieve the right consistency. Let sit about 5 minutes while you heat your skillet to medium heat. Add about 1 tbsp coconut oil. When melted and pan is hot, use a ¼ cup measuring cup and scoop batter onto pan for each pancake. Cook 3 to 5 minutes on first side, or until bottom is golden brown, edges are dry, and bubbles have formed on top. Carefully flip with a flexible spatula, then cook another 2 to 3 minutes on second side.

I once had a pancake party and made a bunch of different combinations. Below are some of my favorites, but feel free to experiment and be as creative as you want.

VARIATIONS:

Pumpkin Pecan Pie: Add 2 tbsp pumpkin puree, ½ tsp cinnamon, ¼ tsp allspice, and ½ cup chopped pecans.

Apple Cinnamon Walnut: Add one cored and peeled apple sliced into 1-inch pieces, ½ tsp cinnamon, ½ cup chopped walnuts.

Banana Chocolate Chip: Add one peeled and sliced banana cut into ¼-inch slices and ½ cup vegan chocolate chips.

Blueberry Buckwheat: Substitute ½ cup buckwheat flour for half of the flour and add 1 cup of fresh or frozen blueberries.

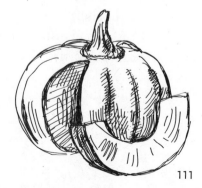

CRANBERRY MUFFINS WITH TOASTED COCONUT ALMOND STREUSEL

(makes 12 muffins)

> These muffins make a delicious breakfast treat or lightly sweet dessert. The crunch of the streusel topping gives the hominess of morning granola, perfect with a cup of coffee. A batch of these also make a good snack for a road trip.

INGREDIENTS

- » 1 ¼ cups brown rice flour
- » ½ cup garbanzo bean flour
- » ½ cup tapioca flour
- » ½ tsp xanthan gum
- » 1 cup organic cane sugar
- » 2 tsp baking powder
- » 1 tsp baking soda
- » 1 tsp sea salt
- » 1 ½ tsp cinnamon
- » ½ cup canola oil
- » ½ cup unsweetened applesauce
- » 1 tbsp ground flax seed mixed with 5 tbsp water
- » ¾ cup unsweetened almond milk
- » 1 tbsp vanilla
- » 1 tsp almond extract
- » 1 cup cranberries

STREUSEL INGREDIENTS

» ¼ cup slivered almonds
» 3 tbsp organic cane sugar
» ¼ cup brown rice flour
» ¼ cup shredded coconut
» 1–2 tbsp melted coconut oil

Preheat oven to 350°F. Combine Streusel ingredients in a small bowl until ingredients clump together, then set aside. In a large bowl, whisk together brown rice flour, garbanzo flour, tapioca starch, xanthan gum, sugar, baking powder, baking soda, sea salt and cinnamon. In a separate bowl, combine oil, applesauce, flax seed mixture, almond milk, vanilla and almond extracts and whisk together. Stir wet ingredients into dry ingredients until batter is smooth and thick. Carefully fold in cranberries. Line muffin tins with papers. Using a ¼ cup measuring cup, scoop batter into the papers. Sprinkle about 1 tbsp of streusel topping over each muffin and lightly press down to ensure topping adheres to batter. Bake for 30 to 35 minutes or until tops are springy and sides of muffins are lightly browned. Cool for 5 to 10 minutes in the pans, then transfer to cooling rack to continue cooling completely.

LOADED OATMEAL

(serves 4)

> This recipe is loaded with fiber, protein, and flavor from the variety of add-ins. Oatmeal is so easy to veganize that your loved ones won't even notice the difference.

INGREDIENTS

» 3 cups of water
» 1 cup vegan milk (I like unsweetened almond)
» 2 cups rolled oats
» ½ cup organic sugar
» ¼ tsp sea salt
» 1 tsp vanilla

Place water, vegan milk, oats, sugar, and sea salt in a sauce pot and bring to a boil. Lower heat and simmer for about 10 minutes, stirring to prevent sticking. When oats thicken to your desired consistency, stir in vanilla. Serve as is or with a pat of vegan margarine and a generous drizzle of real maple syrup. You can also have fun with the following variations:

Apple Walnut: Peel and core one apple and dice into 1-inch pieces. Add to pot along with ½ tsp of cinnamon. When oatmeal is done, stir in ½ cup chopped walnuts.

Cinnamon Sugar: Sprinkle the top of your oatmeal with 2 tbsp brown sugar and a shake or two of cinnamon.

Banana Chocolate: Peel and slice banana into ½-inch slices and cook along with the oatmeal. When oatmeal is

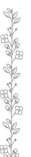

done, remove from heat then stir in ½ cup vegan chocolate chips.

Pina Colada: Use one can of coconut milk in place of the vegan milk and stir in ½ cup dried pineapple cut into ½-inch pieces.

Superfood: Top each bowl of oatmeal with ¼ tsp turmeric, ¼ tsp cinnamon, 1 tbsp ground flax seed, 1 tbsp hemp seed, ¼ cup dried cranberries, ¼ cup chopped walnuts, 8 blackberries, and 1 sliced banana, with extra almond milk and a drizzle of maple syrup.

PINA COLADA CONGEE

(serves 4)

> Congee is an Asian rice pudding that can be made savory or sweet. It's a nice creamy breakfast alternative to oatmeal or a lightly sweet dessert. I like this combination of flavors, but feel free to experiment with your favorite fruits or veggies.

INGREDIENTS

» 1 cup jasmine rice
» 4 dried pineapple rings chopped into ½-inch chunks (about 1 cup)
» ¼ cup organic sugar
» pinch of sea salt
» 1 15 oz. can coconut milk
» 2 cups water
» ¼ cup dried shredded coconut (for garnish)

In a 3 qt. sauce pot, combine all ingredients except dried coconut. Cover and bring to a boil, then lower heat and cook 30 to 40 minutes, or until rice and pineapple pieces have softened. There should still be liquid in the pot. Gently stir rice with the coconut liquid to make a creamy porridge, adding more water if necessary. In a small pan set on medium heat, toast shredded coconut for 3 to 5 minutes, or until lightly browned. Ladle congee into four bowls and top with toasted coconut.

OLD-FASHIONED BANANA BREAD

(yield: 1 loaf)

> This is a super dense and moist bread that tastes great with your morning chai tea or as an afternoon snack at the office.

INGREDIENTS

» 1 ¾ cup all purpose flour (or substitute 1 cup gluten-free flour, ¾ cup brown rice flour, plus ½ tsp xanthan gum)
» 1 tsp baking soda
» ½ tsp baking powder
» ½ tsp salt
» ½ tsp cinnamon
» 2 tbsp ground flax seed plus ⅓ cup water
» 3 very ripe bananas, mashed
» 1 cup organic sugar
» ½ cup canola oil (or substitute ½ cup applesauce to make it oil-free)
» 1 tsp vanilla
» ½ cup chopped walnuts or pecans

Preheat oven to 350°F. Grease and flour a large loaf pan. In a large bowl, mix together flour, baking soda, baking powder, salt, and cinnamon. In a food processor, pulse together flax seed mixture, bananas, sugar, canola oil (or applesauce), and vanilla until creamy with just a few small bits of bananas remaining. Add wet mixture to dry and stir together until no dry lumps of flour remain. (The batter will be thick, but don't worry!) Fold in nuts. Spread into prepared pan, making the edges and corners higher than in the center. Bake for 40 to 50 minutes or until top is browned and a toothpick inserted in the center comes out clean. Let cool in pan 20 minutes. Use a knife to gently loosen bread from sides of pan, then invert onto a cooling rack. You'll want to dive right in, but be patient and let cool completely before cutting.

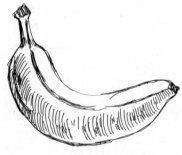

BUCKWHEAT GALETTE WITH SPINACH, MUSHROOM, AND FENNEL SEED

(serves 4)

A galette is a savory crepe that's naturally gluten-free because it's made with buckwheat flour. This thin pancakes can be filled with any sautéed vegetables or eaten plain with a sauce. I enjoyed this combination at Delice & Sarrasin, a French vegetarian bistro in New York. It's a little bit complicated to master the perfect crepe at first, but the effort will be worth it.

INGREDIENTS

» 1 cup buckwheat flour
» 1 tsp sea salt
» 1 ¾ cups water (approx.)
» 1 tbsp ground flax seed mixed together with 3 tbsp water
» 1–2 tbsp coconut oil

FILLING INGREDIENTS

» 1 tbsp olive oil
» 8 oz. button or cremini mushrooms, sliced thinly
» 10 oz. baby spinach
» 1 shallot, peeled and thinly sliced
» 1 clove garlic, minced finely
» ¼ tsp fennel seeds
» ¼ tsp sea salt
» fresh cracked black pepper

Mix flour and salt together in a large bowl. Gradually add 3 cups of water one cup at a time, stirring well after each addition. Whisk in flax mixture until well combined. Cover batter and refrigerate 1 to 2 hours. Meanwhile, in a large skillet on medium heat, sauté sliced mushrooms and shallots 3 to 5 minutes, or until mushrooms are lightly browned. Add baby spinach, cover, and let cook another 3 to 5 minutes or until spinach has wilted. Remove cover, add one clove of minced garlic and fennel seeds, and let cook 3 to 5 minutes, or until water has evaporated. Stir mixture together and season with salt and pepper. Place spinach mixture in a bowl and cover while preparing crepes.

Remove galette batter from the refrigerator and check for consistency, which should be thin and pourable. Stir in remaining ⅓ cup of water if necessary. Heat a large skillet on medium high heat and test with a drop of water to see if it's ready. If the water sizzles, your pan is hot enough. If it's too hot, lower heat to medium. Add 1 tbsp coconut oil to pan and spread it around to melt and coat pan evenly. Ladle about ½ cup of batter into pan and swirl it around to thinly coat bottom of pan. Cook for 1-2 minutes on the first side until the bottom is golden and lifts easily from the pan. Gently flip with a spatula and cook the second side for another minute or two. Transfer cooked crepe to a plate and cover with a towel to keep warm. Continue with remaining crepes, adding coconut oil as necessary to prevent sticking. Evenly divide spinach and mushroom mixture and place in the center of each crepe. Fold over four ends of crepe into the center to form a square galette. Top with a dollop of Dijon Crema.

TOFU FLORENTINE QUICHE

(serves 6 to 8)

> This was a big hit at my New Year's Day Vegan Brunch, and everyone raved that you'd never know this quiche was vegan. It's delicious eaten warm right out of the oven or cold straight from the fridge.

INGREDIENTS

» 1 tbsp olive oil
» ½ cup onion
» 1 clove garlic
» 1 lb. block extra firm tofu
» 1 tbsp umeboshi vinegar
» 1 tbsp fresh lemon juice
» 1 tbsp nutritional yeast
» 1 tsp sea salt
» 2 tbsp water (approx.)
» 4 oz. Daiya cheddar shreds
» 8 oz. frozen chopped spinach (thawed)
» 2 tbsp sesame seeds
» 1 frozen vegan pie crust

Preheat oven to 350°F. In a large skillet on medium heat, sauté onion and garlic in olive oil until softened and beginning to brown, about 5 to 7 minutes. Transfer to a food processor along with crumbled tofu, vinegar, lemon juice, nutritional yeast, and sea salt. Blend together adding a tbsp or two of water until texture is thick and spreadable, but not too smooth. Add half of the Daiya and all of the spinach, pulsing together to combine. Prick the bottom of the pie crust lightly with a fork, then pour the filling into the crust, spreading it evenly. Spread the remaining shredded cheese over the top then sprinkle sesame seeds around the circumference. Bake for 20 to 25 minutes, then another 10 minutes at 400°F to melt cheese.

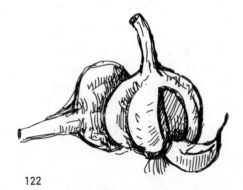

RAW OVERNIGHT BANANA BERRY CHIA PUDDING

(serves 2 to 4)

> If you like the creaminess of pudding but don't want all the calories and hassle of cooking over a stovetop, this recipe for raw chia pudding will win you over. Assemble it in covered mason jars the night before and have a grab-and-go breakfast ready in the morning as everyone rushes off to school and work.

INGREDIENTS

» 2 cups almond milk
» 4 tbsp agave syrup
» 1 tsp vanilla
» 1 ripe banana
» pinch of sea salt
» ⅔ cup chia seeds
» fresh sliced strawberries, banana, and blueberries for garnish

In a high speed blender, puree together almond milk, agave syrup, vanilla, banana, and sea salt until smooth. Pour into large bowl, then stir in chia seeds and let sit for at least an hour, stirring occasionally to prevent the seeds from sticking together. The mixture will start watery, but then get gelatinous like tapioca pudding the longer it sits. This can be refrigerated overnight, though you may need to add more almond milk if it's too thick in the morning. Garnish with fruit such as sliced banana and fresh berries or layer in a parfait cup with a dollop of Coconut Whip on top.

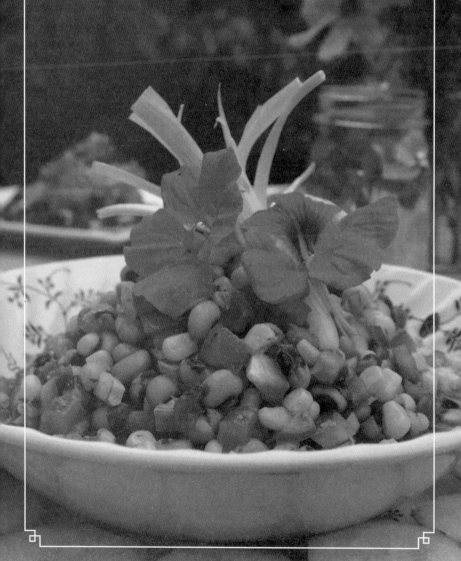

Lunch

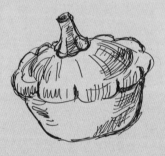

Lunch

While I tend to make lunch my big meal of the day, often eating around 2 or 3 o'clock in the afternoon when I've finished cooking for clients, I know that isn't how most people eat. Instead, lunch is a quick meal squeezed in between meetings and the busy work day. I get that. A soup, salad, sandwich, or a snack is often what will suffice to tide us over until the end of the work day. That's why I've compiled this list of recipes that are portable, easy to make at home, and require little preparation for a meal at the office behind the computer, because I know that's the reality of our fast-paced lives. Keep these guidelines in mind when preparing lunch for yourself and your family so that no one resorts to a bag of potato chips when hunger strikes in the middle of the day.

Make it portable.
A sandwich, pita pocket, or a wrap are handy little containers for a meal.

Leftovers make a good lunch.
Make an extra serving or two for dinner, than pop the leftovers into a container for lunch the next day.

Easy assembly.
A salad that comes together in a minutes with only a few ket ingredients takes little time to prepare the night before.

Ready to eat and enjoy.
Use a tiffin or compartmentalized bento box for storing and transporting meals that don't require any heating

Tasty and satisfying.
A small meal packed with flavor and fiber will satisfy you through dinner time.

Salads

TRI-COLOR SLAW

(serves 2 to 4)

> Make this colorful salad for a picnic buffet or as a side with Barbecue Jackfruit Sliders. It's a tasty, crunchy, and satisfying summer treat.

INGREDIENTS

- » ½ cup vegan mayonnaise
- » 2 tbsp apple cider vinegar
- » 1 tsp agave syrup
- » 1 tsp garlic powder
- » ½ tsp sea salt
- » 1 cup shredded green cabbage
- » 1 cup shredded purple cabbage
- » 2 carrots, peeled and ends removed

Using a box grater or food processor, shred green and purple cabbage and carrots. Mix vegan mayonnaise, vinegar, and agave together in a small bowl. In a separate bowl, combine shredded cabbage and carrot, and briefly squeeze together to soften. Pour dressing on top and mix well. Refrigerate to allow flavors to blend.

MEDITERRANEAN QUINOA SALAD

(serves 4 to 6)

This recipe is super simple and is loaded with flavor. I love using lacinato kale, but I've also substituted fiddlehead ferns when they're in season. Garnish this pretty salad with toasted pine nuts and herb blossoms of chive, oregano, or basil during the summer.

INGREDIENTS

» 1 bunch lacinato kale (approximately 10 to 12 leaves, stems removed), chopped
» ¼ cup olive oil
» ½ cup diced shallot
» 2–3 cloves garlic, minced (to taste)
» 10 sun-dried tomatoes in oil, cut into strips (or use dry sun-dried tomatoes and soak in water)
» ½ cup kalamata olives, sliced in half
» ¼ cup toasted pine nuts
» 2 cups cooked quinoa
» 2 tbsp lemon juice
» approx. ½ tsp sea salt (to taste)
» ¼ tsp coarsely ground black pepper

Heat the oil in a large, deep pan over medium heat and sauté the shallots in the hot oil until soft. Add the garlic and keep sautéing until the shallots begin to turn light golden. Stir in the kale, sun-dried tomatoes, and olives and cook until kale has wilted, about 5 minutes. Turn off heat and combine in a large bowl with quinoa, lemon juice, salt, and pepper. Gently stir together. Taste for balance and adjust seasonings if desired. Let cool, then refrigerate at least a half an hour before serving.

Note: For perfectly fluffy quinoa, start with 1 cup of quinoa (rinsed and drained) and 1 ½ cups water in a sauce pot. Cover pot, bring to a boil, then reduce heat to low. Cook for 15 minutes, then remove saucepan from heat and let sit for 5 minutes. Uncover and fluff gently. Using this method, 1 cup of raw quinoa yields about 1 ½ to 2 cups cooked.

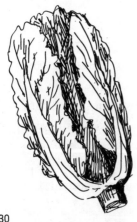

WARM WALNUT, CARROT, SNOW PEA, AND BROWN RICE SALAD

(serves 4)

This is a great way to use up leftover rice. It can be eaten warm like a stir-fry or cooled and served on a bed of shredded Savoy cabbage for lunch. I also like scooping it up with raw stalks of bok choy, but you can use chopsticks if you prefer.

INGREDIENTS

» ½ cup walnuts, roughly chopped
» 1–2 tbsp peanut oil
» 2 carrots, peeled and sliced at an angle into 1/4 inch rounds
» 1 cup snow peas, ends and strings removed
» 1 scallion, sliced thin
» 1 clove garlic, pressed through a garlic press
» 1" piece of fresh ginger, pressed through a garlic press to release juices
» 2 tbsp mirin
» 2 cups cooked brown rice
» 2 tbsp tamari
» 2 tsp agave syrup
» 1 tbsp rice vinegar
» 2 tsp toasted sesame oil
» sea salt

In a large skillet on medium heat, toast walnuts for 1 to 2 minutes or until fragrant. Remove from pan, then add about a teaspoon or two of peanut oil. Add sliced carrots and a pinch of sea salt, then spread them evenly in the pan. Cook for 1 to 2 minutes, or until bright orange. They should be firm but not crisp. Remove from pan, then add another teaspoon of oil, snow peas, and a pinch of salt. Spread them out evenly and let cook for 1 to 2 minutes or until bright green. Remove from pan, add another teaspoon of oil, scallions, garlic, and ginger. Let cook for 1 to 2 minutes or until fragrant, then deglaze with mirin. Gently fold in brown rice, making sure to break apart any clumps. In a mug or small bowl, stir together tamari, agave syrup, vinegar, and toasted sesame oil until well blended. Add to pan and gently fold in cooked vegetables and walnuts. Turn off heat and season to taste. There should be a balance of salty, sweet, spicy, and sour. If flavors seem off, adjust according to what is missing.

WORLD PEAS SALAD

(serves 4 to 6)

> I once catered a bridal shower where one of the guests was telling me about a family favorite salad called "Carolina Caviar," which she enjoyed when growing up in the south. I asked her what was in it and, with the exception of Caesar dressing which is made with anchovies, the ingredients were vegan. She proudly referred to it as "Redneck Caviar," but I decided to change the name to make it a bit more inclusive.

SALAD INGREDIENTS

» 1 15 oz. can black-eyed peas, drained and rinsed
» ½ cup sweet red bell pepper, finely diced
» ½ cup green bell pepper, finely diced
» 1 tbsp jalapeno, finely diced
» 10 oz. frozen yellow corn, drained and thawed
» 2–3 scallions, finely sliced
» ½ cup cilantro, finely chopped
» ½ of a 15 oz. can of diced tomatoes

DRESSING INGREDIENTS

» ¼ cup apple cider vinegar
» ¼ cup olive oil
» 1 tsp agave syrup
» 1 clove garlic, minced
» ½ tsp sea salt
» a few splashes of hot sauce

Combine all of the salad ingredients in a large bowl. In a separate bowl, whisk together all of the dressing ingredients. Combine dressing with the salad ingredients, season with salt and hot sauce, then refrigerate at least a half an hour before serving. Garnish with fresh cilantro or scallions.

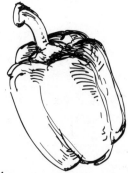

SHAVED BRUSSELS SPROUT SALAD

(serves 4)

> I like to think of this salad as a "spring slaw" for the spring thaw, but it's also nice in the fall when crisp apples are in season. The bright greens contrast with pops of color from red cranberries, making it a perfect seasonal transition that's loaded with antioxidants that will boost the immune system and fight off those colds and flus. .

SALAD INGREDIENTS

- » 1 pound Brussels sprouts, trimmed, thinly shaved
- » 1 organic Honeycrisp apple, cut into wedges and thinly sliced into matchsticks
- » 1 endive, thinly sliced into half moons
- » 2–3 large leaves lacinato kale, ribs removed, thinly sliced into ribbons
- » ½ cup dried cranberries
- » ½ cup toasted pecans, chopped

DRESSING INGREDIENTS

- » 1 tbsp lemon
- » 1–2 tbsp agave syrup
- » 1 tbsp apple cider vinegar
- » 2–3 tbsp extra virgin olive oil
- » ⅛ tsp sea salt

Cut off and discard stem ends of Brussels sprouts. Using a food processor with shredding blade, drop Brussels sprouts into the shoot to thinly shave them. Transfer to a large bowl and add apple, kale, endive, cranberries and pecans. In a separate bowl, whisk lemon juice, agave, cider vinegar, olive oil and salt, until completely blended. Pour over salad mixture and toss gently to mix.

Note: Shaved Brussels sprouts, sliced kale, and endive can be combined ahead of time, stored in a ziplock bag, or covered and stored in fridge. When ready to serve, simply toss with remaining ingredients.

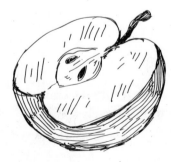

GREEK LENTIL AND BROWN RICE SALAD WITH LEMON AND OLIVES

(serves 4 to 6)

> I love this salad in the summer when my perennial oregano starts taking over the garden. The combination of lemon and green herbs is refreshing on a hot afternoon.

INGREDIENTS

- » 4 tbsp olive oil, divided
- » 1 carrot, peeled and finely diced
- » 1 small onion, finely chopped
- » 2 garlic cloves, minced
- » 1 ¼ cups dried French lentils
- » 2 ½ cups water
- » 1 bay leaf
- » 1 cup long-grain brown rice
- » ½ cup pitted kalamata olives, sliced
- » ½ cup fresh Italian parsley, chopped
- » 2 tbsp fresh oregano, chopped
- » 2 tbsp lemon juice
- » 2 tsp finely grated lemon peel
- » Salt and freshly ground black pepper

Heat 1 tbsp of oil in a large saucepan. Add the carrot, onion, and garlic and sauté until the onion is translucent, about 5 minutes. Stir in the lentils. Add 2 ½ cups of water and bay leaf and bring to a boil over high heat. Decrease the heat to medium-low., cover, and simmer gently until the lentils are just tender, about 15 to 20 minutes. Drain excess water, then transfer the lentils to a large bowl.

Meanwhile, place rice in a sauce pot with 2 cups water, cover, and bring to a boil over high heat. Lower heat and simmer until the rice is tender and the liquid is absorbed, about 25 to 30 minutes (do not stir the rice as it cooks). Fluff the rice with a fork and transfer to the bowl with the lentils. Add the olives, parsley, oregano, lemon juice, and lemon peel. Toss the mixture with the remaining 3 tbsp olive oil to coat. Season, to taste, with salt and pepper. Serve warm or refrigerate for a cold salad.

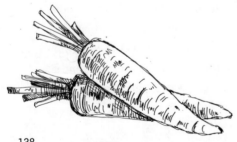

Soups

CURRIED RED LENTIL SOUP

(serves 4)

> This is a satisfying soup that comes together quickly and is oh so satisfying on a cold and dreary day. The flavors will perk you up, and the spices combined with ginger, garlic, and lemon will boost your immune system. At the first sign of a cold, whip up a big pot and you'll feel healthy in no time.

INGREDIENTS

» 1 onion, diced
» 1 clove garlic, minced
» 2-inch slice of fresh ginger, minced
» 1 ½ cups red lentils
» 4 cups water
» 1 tsp turmeric
» 2 tsp curry powder
» 1 tsp sea salt
» ½ cup coconut milk (from can)
» juice of 1 lemon (about 2–3 tbsp)
» chopped cilantro or scallion for garnish (optional)

Place onion, garlic, ginger, lentils, turmeric, curry powder, and water in a large sauce pot, cover, and bring to a boil. Lower heat and simmer gently for 20 to 30 minutes until the lentils are soft. Stir in coconut milk and lemon juice and season with sea salt. You may need to adjust the water depending on the consistency, which should be smooth and creamy not thick and gloppy. Once the correct consistency is achieved, garnish with fresh cilantro or scallion just before serving.

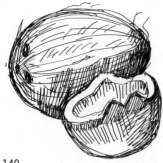

BERBERE SPICED LENTILS WITH LEMON & SPINACH

(serves 4 to 6)

> Berbere is a spice blend used in Ethiopian cooking. A little goes a long way, so if you're hesitant about too much heat, start with a little and gradually add more to suit your taste. It's very warming, as a soup should be, so if you crave heat, feel free to double my recommended amount.

INGREDIENTS

» 1 tbsp unrefined coconut oil
» 1 medium onion, peel removed and diced
» 2 stalks of celery, ends removed and diced
» 2 large carrots, peeled and cut into ¼ inch half moons
» 2 cloves garlic, minced
» 1 large russet potato, cut into ½ inch dice (about 1½ cups)
» 1 cup dry French lentils, rinsed and picked over
» ½ cup dry brown lentils, rinsed and picked over
» 5–6 cups water
» ½ tsp garlic powder
» 1–2 tsp Berbere spice (or substitute 1–2 tsp smoked paprika plus ¼ tsp cayenne pepper)
» ½ tsp coriander
» ¼ tsp oregano
» ¼ tsp black pepper
» 2 tbsp tomato paste
» 1 tbsp fresh lemon juice
» ½ tsp apple cider vinegar
» 2 tsp salt
» 8 oz. frozen chopped spinach, thawed and squeezed dry

Heat olive oil in a large heavy-bottomed soup pot over medium heat. Add onion, celery, and carrots, and sauté until softened, about 5 to 10 minutes. Add garlic, diced potato, lentils, and 5 cups of water. Stir together, cover, and bring to a boil. Once soup has reached a boil, reduce heat to low and simmer covered for 30 minutes. Stir in garlic powder, Berbere spice, coriander, oregano, black pepper, tomato paste, lemon juice, vinegar, and salt. Check for seasoning, then stir in chopped spinach until wilted. Add more water if the soup is too thick and season to taste.

Variations: I like to make a big batch of lentils on the weekend that can be modified throughout the week by adding different flavor combinations. Start by doubling the basic lentil recipe, but hold off on adding the Berbere and coriander. This way you can modify the spices based on the Flavor Burst Guide and vary your meals throughout the week.

For example, on Day 1 start with the basic lentils and serve them with brown rice. On Day 2, take a scoop of the lentils and mix with a can of fire-roasted tomatoes and a handful of fresh chopped basil and parsley and serve as a vegan bolognese sauce over pasta. On Day 3, take a scoop of lentils and sauté in a pan with chili powder, cumin, and fire-roasted tomatoes to make a Mexican chili that can be served with brown rice and avocado. On Day 4, take a scoop of lentils and sauté in a pan with turmeric, curry powder, ginger and garlic, then add coconut milk, chopped spinach, and a squeeze of lemon to make a curry with basmati rice. On Day 5, scoop the lentils into green bell peppers, top with Daiya shredded cheese, and bake covered in a 400 degree oven for 40 to 50 minutes to make stuffed peppers. On Days 6 and 7, use the lentils as a filling for a galette, topping on tostada, wrapped in a tortilla like a burrito, or combined with leftover brown rice and formed into a lentil loaf or patties. Experiment and have fun!

GARDEN VEGGIE SOUP

(serves 4 to 6)

> This is my summer harvest go-to soup when the farmers markets are so overstocked with zucchini they're practically giving them away. Use whatever veggies are in abundance in your garden.

INGREDIENTS

» 2 tbsp olive oil
» 1 small yellow onion, diced (about 1 cup)
» 1 stalk of celery, ends trimmed and cut into ¼ inch dice (about 1 cup)
» 2 carrots, peeled and cut into ¼ inch half moons (about 1 cup)
» 2 cloves garlic, minced finely
» 2 zucchini, cut into ¼-inch half moons (about 2 cups)
» 1 yellow squash, cut into ¼-inch half moons (about 1 cup)
» 1 cup string beans, ends trimmed and cut into 1 inch pieces
» 4–5 cups water
» 2 Tbsp nutritional yeast
» 2 tsp finely chopped fresh oregano (or substitute dried)
» 2–3 Tbsp fresh lemon juice
» 2 tsp sea salt

In a large pot sauté onion, celery and carrot in olive oil until soft. Add a couple cloves of minced garlic and sauté another minute. Add zucchini, yellow squash, green beans, and enough water to cover (about 4 to 5 cups). Bring to a boil, cover, then lower heat and simmer for about 20 to 30 minutes or until veggies are soft and beginning to fall apart. Stir in nutritional yeast, oregano, the juice of ½ a lemon, and sea salt. Garnish with fresh oregano or seasonal herb.

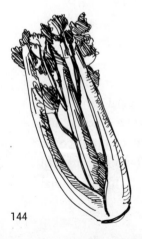

BUTTERNUT SQUASH BISQUE

(serves 4 to 6)

> This is a smooth and rich soup that guests will never suspect is vegan. I like serving it in the fall topped with toasted pepitas as a crunchy contrast.

INGREDIENTS

- » 1 tbsp olive oil
- » 1 cup yellow onion, chopped
- » 1 clove garlic, minced
- » 1 cup garnet yam, peeled and cut into 2-inch cubes
- » 2 large carrots, peeled and cut into 2-inch pieces
- » 2 cups butternut squash, peeled and cut into 2-inch cubes
- » 2 cups of water
- » 1–2 cups almond milk
- » 2 tbsp mellow white miso
- » 1 tsp sea salt
- » 1 scallion, sliced fine

In a large pot, sauté onion and garlic in olive oil until translucent. Add yam, carrots, parsnip, squash and enough water to cover (approximately 2 cups), and bring to a boil. Cover pot, lower heat, and simmer approximately 15 to 20 minutes, or until vegetables are fork-tender. Turn off heat and let cool 10 to 15 minutes. Place cooled vegetables and miso in blender and puree with enough almond milk to make mixture smooth and creamy (approximately 2 cups). If soup is too thick, add more almond milk. Season with sea salt. Return pureed soup to pot and simmer over low heat before serving. Garnish with fresh scallions and toasted pepitas.

ROOTSY CHOWDER

(serves 4 to 6)

> This is another warming soup I love eating during cold weather. Make a big batch on the weekend then enjoy it all week. It gets thicker the longer it refrigerates.

INGREDIENTS

» 2 tbsp olive oil
» 1 small yellow onion, diced (about 1 cup)
» 1 stalk of celery, ends trimmed and cut into ¼ inch dice (about 1 cup)
» 2 carrots, peeled and cut into ¼ inch half moons (about 1 cup)
» 2 cloves garlic, minced finely
» 1 parsnip, peeled and cut into ¼ inch half moons (about 1 cup)
» 1 large jewel yam, peeled and cut into 1 inch cubes (about 3 cups)
» 1 medium turnip, peeled and cut into 1 inch cubes (about 2 cups)
» 5–6 cups water
» 1 cup raw cashew pieces
» 2–3 tbsp nutritional yeast
» 2–3 tbsp fresh lemon juice
» 2 tsp sea salt

In a large pot sautée onion, celery and carrot in olive oil until soft, then add a couple cloves of minced garlic, parsnip, yam, turnip, and enough water to cover (about 5 cups). Bring to a boil, cover, then lower heat and simmer for about 30 to 40 minutes or until veggies are soft and beginning to fall apart.

Meanwhile, soak raw cashews in water for half an hour or longer, then drain and rinse them in a colander. Scoop about 4 cups of cooked veggies and broth and place in blender along with soaked cashews, nutritional yeast, and juice of ½ a lemon. Blend till smooth, then stir into soup and season with sea salt.

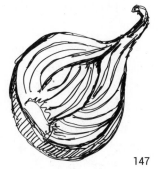

Sandwhiches & Wraps

BARBECUE JACKFRUIT SLIDERS*

(serves 2 to 4)

> You'll love this healthy twist on a summer barbecue favorite which uses young jackfruit in place of pork that's just as flavorful but without all the extra calories and fat. The key is making a good barbecue sauce that balances salty, sweet, savory, and spicy. Start with this basic sauce and vary it according to your tastes by substituting pureed pineapple or mango for the sweet, using lime juice for the sour, or increasing the spicy by adding cayenne or habanero pepper. Enjoy with a crunchy tri-color slaw on Vietnamese Bahn Mi for a tasty meal to go.

*Canned Jackfruit in Brine can be purchased at Asian grocery stores or ordered on-line.

JACKFRUIT DRY RUB INGREDIENTS

- » 20 oz. can of jackfruit in brine (I use Aroy-D brand)
- » 1 tbsp Sucanat
- » 1 tsp paprika
- » ½ tsp garlic powder
- » ½ tsp salt

- » ½ tsp chili powder
- » ¼ tsp black pepper

Drain jackfruit into colander, remove any seed pods, then mix with seasonings in a large bowl.

BARBECUE SAUCE INGREDIENTS

- » 7 oz. tomato paste
- » ½ cup water
- » ½ tsp garlic powder
- » ½ tsp paprika
- » 2 tbsp Dijon mustard
- » 1 tbsp bourbon
- » 2 tbsp tamari
- » 2 tbsp maple syrup
- » 3 tbsp apple cider vinegar
- » 1 tsp Sriracha
- » ½ tsp liquid smoke
- » ¼ tsp sea salt

Stir all ingredients together in a bowl until smooth, adding water as necessary to achieve pourable consistency.

SAUTÉ INGREDIENTS

- » 1–2 tbsp olive oil
- » 1 cup onion, sliced into half moons
- » 1 clove garlic, minced

In a large pot or skillet set on medium heat, heat oil and sauté onion for several minutes until soft. Add garlic and jackfruit and sauté 5 to 10 minutes, or until lightly browned. Add about ¾ cup of the barbecue sauce and ½ cup water and stir together with jackfruit mixture. Cover pot, bring to a boil, then lower heat and simmer 20 to 25 minutes. Stir mixture every 5 to 10 minutes to prevent sticking and cook until jackfruit has softened and easily pulls apart with a fork. Add a bit more barbecue sauce, then turn up heat to medium high to reduce sauce and concentrate flavors while stirring constantly. Serve with veggie slaw.

Variation: If you don't have jackfruit, substitute tempeh which has been cubed or cut into slices. You could also substitute a 15 oz. can of drained and rinsed chickpeas.

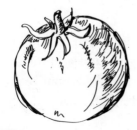

MOCK CHICKEN SALAD

(serves 2 to 4)

> This is a quick and easy "go to" filling for sandwiches and wraps that can easily be made ahead and assembled for the next day's lunch.

INGREDIENTS

- » 20 oz. can of jackfruit in brine, drained and rinsed
- » ½ cup vegan mayonnaise
- » 1 tbsp Dijon mustard
- » 1 tbsp fresh squeezed lemon juice
- » ¼ tsp garlic powder
- » ¼ tsp sea salt
- » 1 stalk celery, diced fine
- » ¼ cup red onion, diced

Bring a large pot of water to a boil. Add jackfruit chunks and boil about 5 minutes, then drain and rinse with cold water until cool to the touch. Squeeze jackfruit over colander to remove excess water and seed pods, then set aside. In a large mixing bowl, whisk together vegan mayonnaise, mustard, lemon juice, garlic powder, and sea salt. Use two forks to shred jackfruit, then combine with dressing and remaining ingredients, mixing lightly until dressing is well incorporated.

Variation: If you don't have jackfruit, substitute tempeh that has been cubed, boiled in water for 5 minutes, drained and squeezed of excess water. You could also use a 15 oz. can of drained and rinsed chickpeas that are mashed with a potato masher. No need to cook the chickpeas.

EGGLESS EGG SALAD

(serves 2 to 4)

> This "familiar to fabulous" vegan alternative to traditional egg salad is a great recipe for a super yummy sandwich spread or salad topper on a picnic buffet. I like making a pretty presentation for parties by placing a scoop of this salad on cucumber rounds or in endive leaves and topping with a sprinkling of finely sliced scallion.

INGREDIENTS

- » ¼ cup green onion, finely sliced
- » 2 stalks celery, finely diced
- » 1 dill pickle, finely diced
- » 1 package of extra firm tofu, drained
- » ½ tsp turmeric
- » ½ tsp sea salt
- » ½ cup vegan mayonnaise
- » 1 tbsp Dijon mustard
- » 1 tsp apple cider vinegar
- » salt to taste

Place green onion, celery, and pickle in a large bowl. Crumble tofu into small chunks on top of veggies. Sprinkle with turmeric and sea salt. Gently stir in vegan mayonnaise, Dijon mustard and apple cider vinegar until color and texture resemble chopped eggs. Add more turmeric if it needs to be more yellow, but be careful not to add too much or it will turn a day-glo hue! Season with salt, as necessary.

FIRE BREATHING DRAGON SALAD
(serves 2 to 4)

If you want a little spicy kick to your sandwiches, this is the tofu salad for you. Slather it on some hearty bread along with ripe tomatoes and crispy green lettuce or add Tri-Color Slaw for an extra crunch.

INGREDIENTS

» 1 lb. tofu
» ¼ cup red onion, finely diced
» 2 tbsp jalapeno, finely diced
» 1 tsp cayenne pepper
» 2 tbsp Dijon mustard
» 2 tsp garlic powder
» 2 tsp horseradish
» 2 tbsp apple cider vinegar
» 2 tbsp dill, minced
» 1 tsp sea salt

Crumble tofu into a food processor fitted with the paddle attachment. Add remaining ingredients and pulse together for about 30 seconds, or until well combined. Scrape down the sides with a spatula and be sure that ingredients are evenly distributed. Pulse several more times if necessary.

Tempeh Tartare on Avocado Toast

(serves 2 to 4)

When fresh herbs are in season, this is a lovely recipe to serve as on an open-faced sandwich for an elegant summer soirée.

INGREDIENTS

- » 8 oz. tempeh, cut into 1-inch cubes
- » 2 tbsp Dijon mustard
- » 3 tbsp olive oil
- » 1 tbsp fresh lemon juice
- » 1 tsp apple cider vinegar
- » ¼ tsp garlic powder
- » ½ tsp sea salt
- » ¼ cup finely chopped Granny Smith apple
- » ¼ cup finely chopped jicama
- » 2 stalks finely chopped celery
- » 2 tbsp finely chopped dill
- » 1 tbsp finely chopped chives (scallion can be substituted)
- » splash of hot sauce
- » 4 lightly toasted slices of bread
- » 1 avocado

Bring a pot of water to a boil and submerge tempeh. Cook for 5 minutes, drain in a colander, and rinse with cold water. Set aside to cool. In a large bowl, whisk together mustard, oil, lemon juice, vinegar, garlic powder, and sea salt. Crumble tempeh into the bowl along with apple, jicama, celery, dill, and chives. Season with sea salt and a splash of hot sauce. Cut avocado in half, then cut each half into 8 thin slices. Lay 4 slices on each piece of toast, then spoon tartare on top. Garnish with fresh herbs or edible flowers.

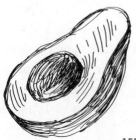

Unfried Beans

(serves 2 to 4)

> This is a simple bean spread that can be used as a sandwich or wrap filling, or spread on a tortilla topped with your favorite vegan cheese and salsa for a quick tostada. I make it fabulous by adding a spoonful of sofritos and a drizzle of Cholula hot sauce.

INGREDIENTS

- » 2 scallions diced
- » ½ cup green bell pepper, diced
- » 2 tbsp jalapeno pepper, diced
- » 1 clove garlic, minced
- » 1 can pinto beans, drained and rinsed
- » 2 tbsp tomato paste
- » 1 tbsp lime juice
- » ½ tsp cumin
- » 1 tsp chili powder
- » 1 tsp sea salt

Place all ingredients into a food processor and pulse together to combine. Blend for about one minute into a paste-like consistency similar to refried beans or a thick hummus and all ingredients have been incorporated. Season to taste.

For Tostada: Preheat oven to 375°F. Place four tortillas on a baking sheet and spread about ¼ of the bean mixture evenly over each. Top each with about ¼ cup salsa and your favorite vegetable topping (I like chopped green peppers or kale). Lay about 2 oz. of shredded vegan cheese on top and bake in the oven for 10 to 15 minutes, or until cheese has melted and tortilla is golden brown and beginning to crisp. Remove from oven and top with a couple spoonfuls of sofrito or sliced avocado.

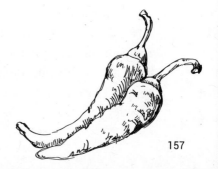

Portobello Pate

(serves 4 to 6)

> This recipe is loaded with protein and savory umami, which makes a satisfying meat alternative. It's a nice as a sandwich spread, salad topper, or dip for crudités. Alternatively, it can be placed into pastry bag and piped onto endive leave in shell pattern for a pretty presentation.

INGREDIENTS

» 1 tbsp olive oil
» 12 oz. portobello mushrooms, cleaned and stems removed
» ½ cup onion, diced
» 1 rib celery, diced
» 2–3 garlic cloves, minced
» ½ cup balsamic vinegar
» 4 oz. extra firm tofu
» ½ cup chopped walnuts
» ¼ cup kalamata olives
» 3 tbsp fresh parsley, chopped
» 1 tsp dried oregano
» ½ tsp sea salt
» ¼ tsp fresh black pepper
» 15–20 endive leaves

In a skillet, sauté mushrooms, onion, celery and garlic in oil until soft, about 5 minutes. Deglaze pan with balsamic vinegar and cook another 5 minutes. Place mushroom mixture into food processor with tofu, walnuts, olives, parsley, oregano, salt and pepper. Process until smooth. Chill mixture before serving.

Mediterranean Tofu

(serves 2 to 4)

> Eat this on its own or as a sandwich filling in crispy Italian bread or a tortilla wrap. This is one of my favorite summer picnic lunches.

TOFU MARINADE INGREDIENTS

» 1 lb. extra firm Chinese style tofu
» 2–3 tbsp tamari
» 1–2 tsp toasted sesame oil

Preheat oven to 400°F. Drain and rinse tofu, then cut block in half horizontally. Slice each half into four ¼–inch slices, then marinate in tamari and toasted sesame oil mixture for at least a half hour. Place marinated tofu on an oiled baking sheet and bake 10 to 15 minutes on each side, or until lightly browned and crisp.

FILLING INGREDIENTS

» 1 cup sundried tomatoes (about 10–12)
» ½ cup kalamata olives
» ¼ cup walnuts
» 1-2 cloves garlic
» 1 large handful fresh Italian parsley
» 2 tsp dried oregano
» ½ tsp sea salt
» Fresh black pepper
» ¼ cup extra virgin olive oil

» 8 oz. roasted red peppers, cut into 4 slices
» 16 large leaves of fresh basil

In a food processor, pulse together sundried tomatoes, olives, walnuts, garlic and parsley to roughly chop. Add oregano, sea salt, and black pepper, then blend together, adding enough olive oil to form a thick paste. You may need to scrape down the sides with a spatula and continue pureeing. To assemble, spread filling ingredients on bread and layer baked tofu, roasted red pepper, and fresh basil on top.

Dinner

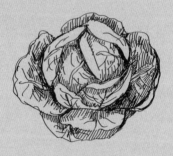

Dinner

Traditional American main courses typically consist of meat, starch, and veggies, with the animal's body part taking the "center of the plate" role. An easy way to "veganize" this format is simply to replace the meat with one of the plant-based substitutes mentioned in the previous chapter. However, if you want to take the familiar and make it fabulous, consider adding a sauce, gravy, or flavor burst from this section which adds interest and variety to an otherwise mundane meal.

Entrees

Pecan Crusted Tempeh

(serves 2 to 4)

> For any diehard meat eater who has never had tempeh, this is the recipe to try. You will convince them that vegan food can be tasty and satisfying and they will never miss "their chicken." I like serving this over mashed root veggies and sautéed greens with Maple Chipotle Crema drizzled over the top or for a ThanksLiving feast with Crimini Mushroom Gravy. Alternatively, it's perfect as a sandwich filling with lettuce, tomato, and spicy brown mustard.

MARINADE INGREDIENTS

» 1 8 oz. package of tempeh, cut into 8 triangle slices
» 2–3 tbsp tamari
» 1 tbsp tomato paste
» 1 tbsp tahini
» 1–2 tsp toasted sesame oil
» enough water to make smooth sauce

TOPPING INGREDIENTS

» ½ cup finely ground pecans
» ½ cup nutritional yeast

» ¼ cup corn starch
» 1 tsp dried oregano
» ½ tsp sea salt

Cut tempeh in half length-wise, then on the diagonal to make four triangles. Stand each triangle on its side and slice in half to make two thin triangles of the same size. Do this with the other triangles so that you have eight thin triangular slices. Stir marinade ingredients together in a large bowl. In a separate bowl, combine topping ingredients. Dip each slice of tempeh into marinade, shaking off excess, then thoroughly coat in topping, pressing to ensure it sticks. Place coated tempeh slices on an oiled baking sheet. Bake at 400°F for 10 to 15 minutes on each side, or until lightly browned and coating is crisp.

Tempeh Stroganoff

(serves 2 to 4)

> This is one of those comfort food favorites that I like eating when the weather gets chilly. For those who miss "their meat," this is a hearty dish loaded with savory umami.

INGREDIENTS

» 1 8 oz. package Lightlife garden vegetable tempeh, cut into 1-inch cubes
» 1 cup frozen peas that have been thawed to room temperature
» 2-3 tbsp olive oil
» 6 crimini or Baby Bella mushrooms, sliced
» 1 shallot, diced fine
» 1 clove garlic, finely minced
» 1 tbsp cornstarch
» 2 tbsp tamari
» 2 cups water
» 1 tbsp tahini
» ½ cup vegan sour cream

Bring a sauce pot of water to a boil and boil tempeh for 5 minutes. Drain in colander and set aside. Meanwhile, heat 1 tbsp oil in skillet on medium heat and add mushrooms and shallot, sprinkling with salt and black pepper. Cook approx. 5 minutes, or until juices are released from mushrooms and they are beginning to brown. Add garlic and cook another minute. In a small bowl, stir together cornstarch, tamari, and water. Pour mixture into sauce pot. Cook over medium heat, stirring constantly until sauce begins to thicken. Remove from heat and quickly whisk in tahini and sour cream to make a creamy sauce. If sauce is too thin, whisk in more tahini. Combine with tempeh and peas and return pan to medium heat to warm thoroughly. Serve over noodles or brown rice.

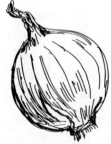

Walnut & Spinach Pesto Stuffed Portobello Caps

(serves 2)

> I like this recipe for summer grilling season. You can assemble the mushrooms on an aluminum foil tray or grill pan and transfer to your grill for cooking to get that nice smoky flavor. It also works well cooked in the oven.

MARINADE INGREDIENTS

» 2 portobello mushrooms, stems removed and reserved
» 2 tbsp balsamic vinegar
» 2 tsp olive oil
» salt and pepper

FILLING INGREDIENTS

» ¼ cup walnuts
» ¼ cup breadcrumbs (gluten-free can be used)
» 8 oz. baby spinach
» ¼ cup fresh chopped parsley
» 1 shallot, diced
» 1 tbsp nutritional yeast
» 1 tsp dried Italian seasoning
» ¼ tsp sea salt

Place portobello mushrooms on baking sheet and drizzle with balsamic vinegar and olive oil, then season with salt and pepper. Bake at 400°F for 10 to 15 minutes, or until soft. Meanwhile, in a food processor, pulse walnuts with breadcrumbs until roughly chopped. Add a handful of spinach, parsley, shallot, reserved mushroom stems, nutritional yeast and salt and pulse together to combine. Place stuffing in mushrooms, top with a sprinkle of breadcrumbs, and return to oven to cook 10 to 15 more minutes, or until warmed through. Sauté remaining spinach in olive oil and place on top of baked mushrooms.

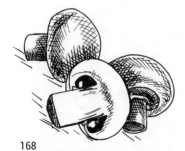

Roasted Eggplant & Tofu Stacks with Fire Roasted Tomato Marinara

(serves 4)

> This is my vegan twist on a traditional Italian favorite of Eggplant Parmesan. The eggplant slices are baked instead of fried and no egg wash is needed with the vegan trick of cornstarch. My Italian relatives raved about it when I served this for Christmas Eve.

COATING INGREDIENTS

- » 2 medium eggplants (about 1 foot long, cut into ½-inch thick slices)
- » 1 cup panko breadcrumbs (or Italian breadcrumbs)
- » 2 tbsp nutritional yeast
- » 2 tsp dried oregano
- » ¼ tsp sea salt
- » fresh black pepper
- » ½ cup unsweetened plain almond milk
- » 1 tsp cornstarch

MARINARA INGREDIENTS

- » 1 20 oz. can of crushed fire-roasted tomatoes
- » 3 cloves garlic
- » ½ cup onion, diced
- » 1–2 tsp dried oregano
- » 1 ½ tsp sea salt

FILLING INGREDIENTS

- » 1 lb. block extra firm tofu
- » juice of half a lemon (about 1–2 tbsp)
- » 1–2 tbsp nutritional yeast
- » 2 cloves garlic
- » 2 tsp dried oregano
- » 1 tsp sea salt, to taste
- » approximately ½ cup plain, unsweetened almond milk
- » 1 handful fresh parsley, chopped
- » 1 8-oz. package of Daiya vegan shredded mozzarella cheese (reserve for topping)

Preheat oven to 400°F. Slice the eggplant in ½--inch rounds. Place on a baking sheet with paper towel underneath and sprinkle with sea salt. Set aside for 30 minutes to allow the moisture to release. Pat dry with paper towel before breading. In a large bowl, mix together breadcrumbs, nutritional yeast, oregano, salt, and pepper. In a separate bowl, mix together cornstarch and almond milk. Dip the eggplant rounds in the almond milk and cornstarch mixture then the breadcrumb mixture, coating both sides evenly. Press the breadcrumbs onto the eggplant and place on oiled baking sheet. Bake the eggplant for 5 to 10 minutes on each side. The eggplant should be browned and slightly crispy when it comes out of the oven. Meanwhile, make sauce by heating a large pot and sautéing onions and garlic in olive oil until soft. Add crushed tomatoes, oregano, and salt, and simmer on low for 10 to 15 minutes. While sauce is simmering, make ricotta filling by crumbling tofu into food processor and pulse together with lemon, nutritional yeast, garlic, oregano and sea salt. You may need to add a little almond milk to make the mixture creamy, but keep a little bit of crumbly texture so that it doesn't become a smooth paste. Once combined, transfer to a bowl and gently stir in chopped fresh parsley.

Assemble: In a 9 × 13 casserole dish, spread ½ cup of the tomato sauce on the bottom of the dish. Place a single layer of breaded eggplant on top of the tomato sauce. Spread dollops of ricotta on top of the eggplant, sprinkle with Daiya mozzarella, then top with another layer of eggplant. Lightly spread tomato sauce on top, reserving some for plating, then sprinkle with Daiya mozzarella. Cover with aluminum foil, then bake at 375°F for 30 to 40 minutes, or until warmed through and cheese is melted.

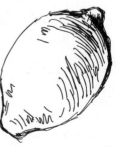

Lasagna with Summer Squash
(serves 8 to 10)

> I was once asked to make lasagna for a bridal shower cooking party with 20 Italian women and only the bride-to-be was vegan. When one of the guests saw the ingredients on the kitchen island, she declared sternly, "Tofu should never be allowed near lasagna." I assured her that the flavors of the sauce and filling were so delicious and authentic tasting she'd never guess she was eating tofu. She hesitantly asked for a small slice to try, then came back a few minutes later, announcing, "I was shocked it tasted so good! I'll have seconds, please."

LASAGNA INGREDIENTS

» 2 (12 oz.) boxes of lasagna noodles (or substitute gluten-free Tinkyada or De Boles noodles)
» 2 zucchini, thinly sliced, blanched in boiling water
» 2 yellow squash, thinly sliced, blanched in boiling water

MARINARA INGREDIENTS

» 3 20 oz. cans of crushed fire-roasted tomatoes
» 3 cloves garlic
» 1 medium onion, diced
» 1–2 tsp dried oregano
» 10–12 leaves fresh basil, chopped
» 1 ½ tsp sea salt

FILLING INGREDIENTS

» 3 1 lb. blocks extra firm tofu
» juice of half a lemon (about 1–2 tbsp)
» 2-3 tbsp nutritional yeast
» 2 cloves garlic
» 2 tsp dried oregano
» 1 tsp sea salt, to taste
» approximately ½ cup almond milk
» 1 handful fresh parsley, chopped
» 2 8 oz. packages of Daiya vegan shredded mozzarella cheese (reserve 1 cup)

Prepare the lasagna noodles according to package directions. Meanwhile, make sauce by sautéing onions and garlic in olive oil until soft. Add crushed tomatoes, oregano, basil and salt, and simmer on low for 10 to 15 minutes. While sauce is simmering, make filling by crumbling tofu into food processor and pulse together with lemon, nutritional yeast, garlic, oregano and sea salt. You may need to add a little almond milk to make mixture creamy, but keep a little bit of crumbly texture so that it doesn't become a smooth paste. Once combined, transfer to a bowl and gently stir in chopped fresh parsley.

Preheat oven to 375°F. Oil the bottom and sides of a 12 × 16 pan, and spread a few spoonfuls of sauce on the bottom. Layer the ingredients in two or three layers, starting with noodles, then tofu ricotta mixture, then Daiya cheese, squash, and sauce. Repeat. End with a layer of noodles and top with Daiya cheese and tomato sauce. Cover with foil, then bake for 50 to 60 minutes, or until bubbly. Uncover and bake 10 to 15 minutes more to melt cheese.

Buffalo Tofu
(serves 2 to 4)

> Eat this as a main course along with Chili Lime Corn on the Cob or serve it as a snack with Cashew Ranch dipping sauce for your next Superbowl party. The basic tofu recipe can be used on its own as a meat substitute without the Buffalo sauce. Experiment with any of the other sauces and gravies in this chapter to add variety to your meals.

MARINADE INGREDIENTS

» 1 16 oz. package of extra firm tofu, cut into 1-inch cubes
» 2–3 tbsp tamari
» 1–2 tsp toasted sesame oil

SAUCE INGREDIENTS

» ½ cup Frank's Hot Sauce
» 1–2 tsp Sriracha
» 1 tsp garlic powder
» 1 tbsp melted vegan margarine

Preheat oven to 400°F. Stir marinade ingredients together in a large bowl and marinate tofu at least 30 minutes. In a separate bowl, mix together sauce ingredients. Place marinated tofu on an oiled baking sheet. Bake for 10 to 15 minutes on each side, or until lightly browned and crisp. Remove from pan and immediate toss with sauce ingredients to coat.

Baked Stuffed Filet of Tofu

(serves 2 to 4)

> If you miss that flavor of the sea, this recipe is the perfect substitute. Make it fabulous by serving it on top of a bed of Garnet Yam Hash and sautéed kale then dolloped with Tartar Sauce. Add a wedge of lemon on the side for garnish.

INGREDIENTS

» 1 lb. block of extra firm tofu
» 2–3 tbsp tamari
» 1–2 tsp toasted sesame oil
» 1 tsp dulse powder
» ¼ cup bread crumbs
» ½ tsp dried parsley
» 2 tsp olive oil
» ¼ tsp sea salt
» fresh black pepper
» 1 tsp fresh lemon juice, plus lemon wedges for garnish

Preheat oven to 400°F. In a large bowl, mix together tamari, toasted sesame oil, and ½ tsp dulse powder. Cut tofu into 2 to 4 long rectangles about 1 inch thick and carefully score the top about ½ inch deep. Submerge tofu in marinade, coating both sides and making sure marinade seeps into scored top. Let marinate for at least a half an hour. In a small bowl, mix together dulse powder, bread crumbs, parsley, olive oil, and sea salt. Place tofu slices on an oiled baking sheet and carefully press breadcrumb mixture into scored tops. Sprinkle with fresh cracked pepper and lemon juice, then bake in oven 35 to 40 minutes, or until bottom has browned and top is dry and beginning to crisp.

Pan-seared Tempeh with Fig & Balsamic Reduction
(serves 2 to 4)

> There is an incredible depth of flavor happening here with salted tempeh, sweet figs, and a rich caramelized vinegar reduction that has a bit of a bite. Roasted Brussels sprouts make a nice pairing for this savory dish.

INGREDIENTS

» 1 8 oz. package tempeh, cut into 8 thin slices
» ¼ cup olive oil
» pinch of sea salt
» fresh cracked black pepper

SAUCE INGREDIENTS

» 1 tbsp olive oil
» 1 shallot, peeled and cut into ¼ inch half moon slices
» ½ cup balsamic vinegar
» ½ cup water
» 1 tbsp agave syrup
» 6 dried Turkish figs, stems removed and cut into quarters
» 1 tbsp vegan margarine
» pinch of sea salt
» crushed black pepper

Cut tempeh in half lengthwise, then each half into two slices so you have four rectangles. Stand each slice on its end and cut laterally so that you have the same sized slices, but half as thick. Heat 2 to 3 tbsp oil in skillet on medium heat, then lay slices in bottom of pan, sprinkling with salt and pepper. Cook approximately 5 minutes on each side, or until golden and crisp, then set aside. Add oil and shallot to the pan and sauté 3 to 5 minutes, or until soft and beginning to brown. Deglaze pan with balsamic vinegar, water, and agave syrup. Add figs, and let simmer approximately 5 minutes, or until sauce begins to thicken and figs are softened. Be careful not to breathe in fumes which can be very pungent! Once sauce thickens, add a pinch of salt and a tbsp of vegan margarine to make glaze, then drizzle over cooked tempeh.

Butternut Squash "Steaks" with Walnut Mushroom Cream Sauce

(serves 2 to 4)

> I like serving this on top of brown rice and sautéed kale for a hearty meal that's satisfying on a chilly autumn evening.

INGREDIENTS

- » 2 tbsp olive oil
- » 1 medium sized butternut squash, peeled, seeds removed, and cut into 8 slices about ½ inch thick
- » ½ cup walnuts, chopped
- » ½ cup yellow onion, diced
- » 8 oz. crimini or button mushrooms, cleaned and sliced
- » 1 tbsp all purpose flour (gluten-free flour or rice flour can be substituted)
- » 1 tbsp nutritional yeast
- » 1 ½ cups water
- » 1 tbsp lemon juice
- » 1 tsp dried oregano
- » ½ tsp sea salt
- » 2 tbsp vegan cream cheese

Preheat oven to 375°F. Place sliced butternut squash slices on an oiled baking sheet and bake for 10 to 15 minutes, or until slightly browned underneath and beginning to soften. Flip over and cook another 5 to 10 minutes. Meanwhile, in a large skillet set on medium heat, heat walnuts until toasted and fragrant, approximately 3 to 5 minutes, then set aside. Add about 1 tbsp of oil to pan and sauté onion for 3 to 5 minutes. Add mushrooms to pan and sauté 5–10 minutes, or until onions and mushrooms are beginning to brown. Add flour and nutritional yeast to pan and stir together with juices to make a roux (paste). Deglaze with water, then stir together with roux to make a thick sauce. Stir in lemon juice and oregano and season with sea salt. Transfer half of the mixture to a high speed blender along with toasted walnuts. Blend together until creamy, adding more water if necessary, then return to pan. Stir in vegan cream cheese, then simmer on low heat until sauce is creamy, adding more water if necessary if sauce becomes too thick. Season with salt and pepper, then pour over butternut squash "steaks."

Baked Stuffed Zucchini Romesco

(serves 2)

> This makes a light meal served on top of a bed of quinoa or penne pasta. Add a drizzle of parsley pistou for a bright, fresh flavor boost.

INGREDIENTS

» 2 medium zucchini, cut in half length-wise
» 1 tbsp olive oil
» 1 cup sundried tomatoes
» 1 cup raw cashews, soaked, drained and rinsed
» 1 clove garlic, crushed
» zest of 1 orange
» juice of 1 orange
» ¼ cup olive oil
» · ¼ cup lemon juice
» 2 tbsp miso
» 2 tsp za'atar spice (or substitute 1 tsp dried oregano)
» 1 tsp sea salt
» fresh black pepper

Scrape the seeds out of the zucchini with a spoon, leaving the walls of each hollowed-out half about ½ inch thick. Drizzle with olive oil and sprinkle lightly with salt and pepper. Bake at 400°F for about 10 minutes, or until beginning to soften. Meanwhile, place all remaining ingredients in food processor and pulse until well combined. Add water if necessary to achieve thick, spreadable paste. Spoon ¼ of the mixture into each zucchini half. Return to oven and bake another 10 to 15 minutes, or until warmed through. Top with a drizzle of Harissa Sauce and/or chopped parsley.

Seared Mushroom "Scallops" with Lemon Caper Sauce

(serves 2)

Served on their own, these make a savory appetizer. The way I like to make them is as a meal by doubling the sauce and serving the mushrooms on top of a bed of wilted spinach tossed with linguini with some French baguette to mop up every last drop.

INGREDIENTS

- » 8 large white stuffing mushrooms, cleaned and stems removed
- » 1 tbsp olive oil
- » ½ tsp Old Bay seasoning
- » 1 clove garlic, finely minced
- » ½ cup plain, unsweetened almond milk
- » 1 tsp corn starch
- » 1 tsp nutritional yeast
- » 1 tsp Dijon mustard
- » 1 tbsp fresh lemon juice
- » 1 tbsp vegan margarine
- » 1 tbsp coarsely chopped fresh parsley
- » 1 tbsp drained capers
- » ½ tsp sea salt

Pour about a tbsp of oil into a skillet on medium heat. Place mushroom caps top side down in skillet, cover, and cook for about 5 minutes, or until golden brown underneath. Flip over, sprinkle each with sea salt and Old Bay Seasoning, and let cook another 5 minutes uncovered, or until juices release. Remove from pan, then add minced garlic and let cook about a minute. Whisk together almond milk, corn starch, nutritional yeast, mustard, and lemon juice, then pour into pan and stir until thickened. Stir in margarine, fresh parsley, capers, and sea salt. Serve Mushroom "Scallops" on top of a bed of wilted baby spinach and linguini and drizzle with lemon caper sauce. For an additional flavor burst, drizzle with parsley pistou.

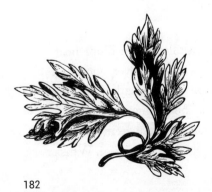

Moroccan Chickpea Tagine
(serves 4 to 6)

> This is a North African stew that has sweet and spicy flavor elements that are addictive. The longer it cooks, the more concentrated the flavors become. Serve with a side of quinoa or millet and top with a dollop of vegan sour cream.

INGREDIENTS

» 1 tbsp olive oil
» 1 small onion, diced
» 3 medium carrots, peeled and sliced into thin rounds
» 1 zucchini, sliced into ½-inch thick half moons
» 3 cloves garlic, minced
» 1 15 oz. can chickpeas, drained and rinsed
» 1 15 oz. can diced tomatoes
» ½ cup water
» ¼ cup dried currants
» 1 tsp turmeric
» 1 tsp smoked paprika
» 1 tsp cinnamon
» ½ tsp cumin
» ¼ tsp cayenne pepper
» 1–2 tsp agave syrup
» 1 ½ tsp sea salt
» 1 handful finely chopped fresh parsley

Heat oil in a large pan over medium heat. Add onion and carrot and sauté 5 to 10 minutes, or until onion is soft and beginning to brown, stirring occasionally. Stir in zucchini, garlic, chickpeas, tomatoes, water, currants, spices, agave syrup, and salt. Cover, bring to a boil, then lower heat and simmer 20 to 25 minutes, stirring occasionally. Add more water if sauce begins to stick or get too thick. Season with sea salt and fresh cracked black pepper and garnish with chopped parsley.

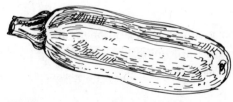

Sides

Zucchini Fritters
(serves 2 to 4)

> I had one of those baseball bat sized zucchinis in my garden and was wondering what to do with it, so I came up with this recipe. I top the fritters with vegan cream cheese, turmeric kraut, and a squeeze of Sriracha, but they're also really good with some ketchup or spicy brown mustard.

INGREDIENTS

- » 1 cup shredded zucchini
- » ½ cup garbanzo bean flour
- » 1 tbsp nutritional yeast
- » ¼ tsp garlic powder
- » ¼ tsp baking powder
- » ¼ tsp sea salt
- » ¼ cup water (approximately)
- » 1-2 tbsp olive oil

Using a box grater, grate the zucchini then place shredded zucchini in a bowl. If you're making a large batch, consider using a food processor on the shredding blade. In a separate bowl, mix together four, nutritional yeast, garlic powder, baking powder, and sea salt, then add enough water to make into a thick paste. Toss zucchini with batter to coat. Heat oil in a large non-stick skillet on media heat. Drop batter in approximately 2 tbsp portions in pan, being careful to leave space between each fritter. Let cook approximately 5 minutes, or until golden brown underneath. Using a spatula, gently flip over each fritter and press down slightly. Let cook another 3 to 5 minutes or until brown and crisp, adjusting the heat if browning occurs too quickly. Remove to a paper towel lined plate.

Black-eyed Pea Fritters
(serves 2 to 4)

> These are a soft and light patty that are nice eaten with a side of Mediterranean Quinoa Salad topped with Horseradish Cashew Mayo. You can also use them as a sandwich filling for a grab-and-go meal.

INGREDIENTS

- 1 15 oz. can of black-eyed peas, drained and rinsed
- 1 tsp garlic powder
- 1 tsp dried oregano
- ½ cup all-purpose flour (rice flour can be substituted)
- ¼ tsp baking powder
- ¼ tsp baking soda
- ½ tsp sea salt
- ½ cup shallots, chopped fine
- ½ cup green pepper, chopped fine
- ½ cup corn starch for dredging
- 2–3 tbsp olive oil for frying

Place all ingredients except corn starch and oil in a food processor and pulse together several times until ingredients begin to blend and stick together. Add a little water if mixture does not come together. When everything has been combined, remove with a spatula and place in a bowl then refrigerate for approximately 30 minutes. Remove mixture from refrigerator and form into patties using a ½ cup measuring ice cream scoop to scoop into equal portions. Flatten to about an inch thick, then lightly dredge in corn starch. Heat a nonstick pan over medium heat and test with a drop of water to be sure it sizzles before adding oil. When hot, add enough oil to thinly coat bottom of pan and fry fritters on medium heat for 5 to 10 minutes on each side, or until lightly browned and crisp.

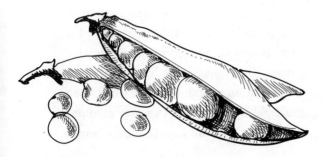

Jamaican Sautéed Black Beans, Greens, and Garnet Yam

(serves 2)

> Serve this dish with some coconut rice for a delicious Caribbean meal. Adjust the heat to your taste with the amount of red chili pepper flakes.

INGREDIENTS

- » 2 large bunches of curly kale, stems removed
- » 1 medium sized garnet yam, peeled and cubed
- » 1–2 tbsp coconut oil
- » 1 cup onion, diced
- » 1 tsp paprika
- » 1 tsp red chili pepper flakes
- » ½ tsp sea salt
- » 1 15 oz. can of diced fire-roasted tomatoes (Muir Glen)
- » 1 15 oz. can of black beans, drained and rinsed

Bring a large pot of water to a boil over high heat. Dip kale in water and blanch for 10 to 15 seconds or until wilted. Remove from pot and rinse in cold water. Remove kale stems, then slice leaves into strips and set aside. Add cubed yam to boiling water and cook 5 to 10 minutes, or until fork tender. Drain, rinse and set aside. Meanwhile, in a large skillet, heat coconut oil on medium heat and sauté onion for 5 minutes, or until lightly browned. Add paprika and chili powder and let cook 30 seconds. Deglaze pan with diced tomatoes and black beans and let cook 5 to 10 minutes. Stir in chopped kale and yam, season with sea salt, and cook another 5 to 10 minutes.

Mashed Root Vegetables
(serves 2 to 4)

This is a versatile recipe, and pretty much any root veggie that's available can be used, except for maybe beets and purple potatoes. Try parsnips, sweet potato, or even celeriac (celery root) and cook until beginning to fall apart to make them easy to mash.

INGREDIENTS

» 1 large Russet potato, peeled and cubed
» 1 garnet yam, peeled and cubed
» 1 turnip, peeled and cubed
» 2 cloves garlic
» 2 tbsp vegan margarine
» ¾ cup unsweetened almond milk
» salt to taste (approximately ½ tsp)

Boil potato, yam, turnip and garlic in a large pot of water for 10 to 15 minutes or until fork tender. Drain and mash together with margarine. Gradually add enough almond milk to whip smooth. Add salt to taste.

Garnet Yam Hash

(serves 2 to 4)

My mom gave me the suggestion for this recipe when I originally said I was going to pan-fry the root veggies and she said, "Why not roast them?" Indeed. Roasting root veggies brings out their natural sweetness, and this hash combines a kick of spice. It's perfect as a base for baked tofu with a sauce drizzled over the top. Thanks, mom!

INGREDIENTS

» 2 parsnips, peeled and ends removed
» 1 carrot, peeled and ends removed
» 1 medium garnet yam, peeled
» 2 tbsp chopped pecans
» ¼ tsp pepper
» ¼ tsp garlic powder
» ¼ tsp cinnamon
» ½ tsp sea salt
» 1 tbsp olive oil

Preheat oven to 400°F. Cut parsnips and carrots in half length-wise, then carefully cut each half down the center. Cut these into ¼-inch thick sticks, then make a stack and cut across to make a ¼-inch dice. Cut yam in half, turn on its flat end, then cut into ½-inch slices. Cut each slice into sticks, then turn and slice into ½-inch dice. Toss diced veggies with pepper, garlic powder, cinnamon, and sea salt. Spread on oiled baking sheet and bake for 25 to 30 minutes, then flip over with spatula and bake another 10 to 15 minutes, or until browned and fork tender.

Meanwhile, heat a skillet on media heat and toast pecans for about 3 to 5 minutes or until fragrant and beginning to brown. Remove veggies from oven and stir in toasted pecans.

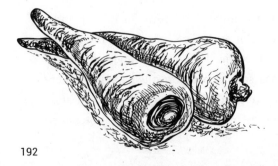

Chili Lime Corn on the Cob
(serves 2 to 4)

This is a twist on Mexican street corn with traditional flavors but without the cotija cheese. If you want a little extra kick, top with maple chipotle crema and chopped cilantro.

Ingredients

» 2 ears of fresh corn, shucked, silk and stem removed, and cut in half
» 1 tbsp vegan margarine
» 1 tbsp nutritional yeast
» 2 tsp chili powder
» ¼ tsp sea salt
» 1 tsp lime juice

Bring a large pot of water to a boil. Carefully place the four pieces of corn into the water and boil for about 5 minutes. Drain into a colander and place on a plate. Spread evenly with vegan margarine, then sprinkle with nutritional yeast, chili powder, and sea salt. Drizzle lime juice over top and press seasonings into corn to coat.

Avocado Fries

(serves 2 to 4)

> While snowed in during a blizzard, I was watching the PBS cooking show, "Moveable Feast," and when the chef made these fries and said they were the most heavenly thing he'd ever tasted, I knew had to try making them. They are, indeed, quite heavenly.

INGREDIENTS

- » 1 cup rice flour
- » ½ teaspoon cumin
- » ¼ tsp chipotle powder
- » ½ tsp sea salt
- » ¼ tsp fresh black pepper
- » ¼ tsp garlic powder
- » ¼ cup water (approximately)
- » 2 tbsp white sesame seeds
- » 1 tbsp black sesame seeds
- » 2 tbsp white quinoa
- » 2 tbsp brown quinoa
- » pinch red pepper flakes
- » 1 avocado, peeled and each cut into 8 slices about 1 inch thick
- » 3–4 tbsp olive oil
- » lemon wedges, to serve

In a small bowl, mix together rice flour, cumin, salt, and pepper. Pour half of it into another bowl. Gradually add water to one of the bowls and whisk together with flour mixture, adding more water as necessary to make a smooth, thin batter. In a third bowl, mix together sesame seeds and quinoa. Dip the avocado slices into the rice flour mixture, then the batter, then coat with the sesame seed mixture, patting down gently to adhere.

Heat the olive oil in a frying pan on medium heat. To test the temperature, drop a small piece of avocado in the oil, which will sizzle and bubble around the edges when hot enough. Fry the avocado slices for about a minute on each side or until the sesame seeds are golden and fragrant. Drain on paper towel and season with salt and pepper. Serve with Tostadas with a garnish of lemon wedges to squeeze over the top.

Sesame String Beans

(serves 2 to 4)

> This is a side dish popular in Szechuan cuisine, a style of cooking originating from Sichuan province in southwestern China which emphasizes the bold flavors of garlic and hot chili peppers. A little heat goes a long way, so modify to your taste!

INGREDIENTS

» 1 tbsp olive oil
» 1 shallot, sliced into half moons
» 1 clove garlic, minced
» ¼ tsp red chili pepper flakes
» 1 lb. string beans, ends trimmed
» 1–2 tbsp tamari
» 1–2 tsp toasted sesame oil
» 1 tbsp sesame seeds

In a large skillet, sauté shallot and garlic in oil on medium heat. When beginning to brown, add red pepper flakes and string beans. Deglaze pan with tamari, then cook 3-5 minutes, stirring frequently. Stir in toasted sesame oil and sesame seeds and cook another 5 minutes or until liquid has been absorbed. The string beans are done when they are beginning to brown and start to squeak, yet still retain some firmness.

Shiitake Bacon
(serves 2)

> Mushrooms add a savory element of umami to any dish, and baking these in the oven will give a nice crispy crunch as well for texture. Use them as a garnish on any pasta or rice dish, or accompanied with a vegetable like Sesame String Beans.

INGREDIENTS

» 6 fresh shiitake mushrooms
» 1 tbsp tamari
» 1 tsp toasted sesame oil
» 1 tsp maple syrup
» ½ tsp apple cider vinegar
» 1 tsp garlic powder
» splash liquid smoke (optional)

Clean shiitake mushrooms, remove stems, and slice into ½ inch wide strips. In a large bowl, mix together remaining ingredients, then toss mushrooms to coat. Let marinate 30 minutes. Preheat oven to 400°F. Evenly distribute marinated mushrooms on an oiled baking sheet, then bake 15 to 20 minutes or until beginning to brown. Flip mushrooms over then bake another 5 to 10 minutes. Mushrooms are done when they're caramelized and slightly crisp with no liquid remaining in the pan.

String Bean Amandine

(serves 2 to 4)

This is a simple side dish that works well when veganizing a plant-based meat-and-potatoes meal. For a variation, Brussels sprouts that have been cut in half and stalk end removed or broccoli florets can be substituted for the string beans.

INGREDIENTS

» 1–2 tbsp olive oil
» 1 shallot, sliced thin
» 1 clove garlic, minced
» 2 tbsp slivered almonds
» 2 cups string beans, ends trimmed, cut in half and blanched
» ½ tsp sea salt

In a skillet on medium heat, sauté shallot in olive oil until golden. Add garlic, slivered almonds and a pinch of sea salt and sauté about a minute. Add blanched string beans and toss together for 2 to 3 minutes or until warmed through. Season with sea salt.

Asian Sesame Cabbage
(serves 2 to 4)

> This is a quick and easy recipe that makes a complete meal when served over rice noodles or ramen with baked tofu and topped with Shiitake Bacon.

INGREDIENTS

» 2 tbsp sesame seeds
» 1 tbsp rice vinegar
» 1 tbsp olive oil
» 4 cups shredded Napa cabbage (green cabbage can be substituted)
» 2 carrots shredded
» 1 tsp toasted sesame oil
» 2 tbsp agave syrup
» 1 tbsp tamari
» ¼ tsp white pepper
» sea salt to taste

In a large skillet, toast sesame seeds over medium heat until golden brown and fragrant, then set aside. Add olive oil to pan and sauté cabbage and carrot for 5 to 7 minutes, or until beginning to wilt. Meanwhile, in a small bowl, mix together vinegar, sesame oil, olive oil, agave syrup, tamari, and pepper. Pour mixture over cabbage and carrots and sauté another 3 to 5 minutes or until blended and veggies have wilted. Top with toasted sesame seeds.

Besan Cakes

(makes 4 cakes)

> This is a simple Indian flatbread that can be served with curry dishes or lentil soup. Perfect for sopping up every last drop

INGREDIENTS

- » 1 cup chickpea (besan) flour
- » 1 tsp baking powder
- » ½ teaspoon cumin
- » ¼ tsp garlic powder
- » ½ tsp sea salt
- » a few grinds of fresh cracked black pepper
- » 2 finely sliced scallions
- » ¾ to 1 cup water (approximately)
- » 2 tsp coconut oil

Whisk all ingredients except oil in a large bowl, adding enough water to make a smooth, thin pourable batter. Let batter sit for about 5 minutes to thicken. Meanwhile, heat a non-stick skillet on medium and add about a teaspoon of coconut oil. When melted, pour about ¼ cup of the batter into the pan. Let cook for about 3 to 5 minutes, or until top gets bubbly and bottom begins to brown. Flip over and cook another minute or two. Transfer to plate and continue cooking the remaining batter, adjusting heat as necessary.

Roasted Asparagus
(serves 2 to 4)

> Roasting is a simple cooking technique to bring out the natural sweetness in vegetables. You can substitute vegetables such as Brussels sprouts cut in half, string beans, or broccoli florets, or use a combination for variety depending on what's in season.

INGREDIENTS

» 1 tbsp coconut oil
» 1 large bunch of asparagus, stem end trimmed
» sea salt

Melt coconut oil then toss with asparagus. Place asparagus on baking sheet and sprinkle with sea salt. Roast in 400°F preheated oven until slightly browned and softened, about 8 to 10 minutes.

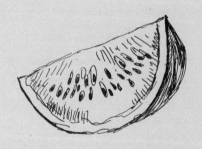

— Sauces and Flavor Bursts —

E ach culture has its own unique blend of herbs and spices that combine together to make its "signature" flavor profile. Most of us are familiar with the heat of cumin, chili powder, and jalapeño pepper common in Mexican food or fresh Mediterranean herbs such as basil, oregano, and parsley found in Italian and Greek cuisine. The ultimate goal is for food to have a balance of SALTY, SWEET, SOUR, and BITTER with a hint of HEAT which create harmony when combined by the creative chef. Any of the sauces in this section can be served on top of baked tofu, pan-fried tempeh, bean cakes and fritters, or any meat substitute.

A sixth flavor element known as UMAMI is essentially a rich, savory quality that makes food satisfying. People who claim they miss "their meat" when they go vegan are actually saying the umami is absent. That can be remedied by adding plant-based ingredients that contain this element, such as mushrooms, tamari (soy sauce), miso (fermented soybean paste), sun-dried tomatoes, or balsamic vinegar.

Over lunch one day at the fantastic vegan restaurant, It's Only Natural in Middletown, Connecticut, the talented vegan chef, Ken Bergeron, told me about his use of "flavor bursts" to liven up dishes. These are concentrated combinations of the four flavor elements unique to each culture (e.g., a garnish of chopped salted peanuts, toasted coconut, lemon zest, and red pepper flakes on top of an Indonesian noodle dish). Use the flavor guide below to add variety to your meals and create your own unique "flavor bursts" to add to recipes.

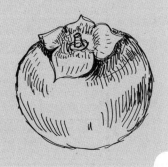

Culture	Prominent flavors & ingredients	Uses
Italian	parsley, basil, oregano, tomatoes, garlic, olive oil	sprinkle fresh herbs over pasts, on pizza, in bean dishes, on risotto, or stir into polenta
Greek	oregano, parsley, Kalamata olives, lemon	stir into bean and rice dishes, in soups and stews
Middle Eastern	oregano, sesame seed, sumac, za'atar, tahini, garlic, lemon, mint, parsley	sprinkle dried herbs on flatbread, stir into soups, add to tofu marinade, season lentils
Mexican	cumin, chili powder, jalapeno, tomatoes, lime, cilantro	mix with rice and bean dishes, guacamole, salsa
Latin American	onion, garlic, chili peppers, tomatoes	sauté as a base for rice and bean dishes
African	cinnamon, turmeric, cloves, cumin, fenugreek, berbere, harissa, garlic, ginger, onions, mint, parsley, sesame seeds	sauté veggies as a base, then mix spices into rice and bean dishes, stir into soups and lentils
Indian	turmeric, curry powder, garam masala, cumin, mustard seed, cardamom, fenugreek, ginger, garlic, coconut oil	sauté garlic, onion, and ginger in coconut oil as a base for lentils and bean dishes, then add tomato paste and spices, finish with coconut milk
Japanese	tamari (soy sauce), garlic, ginger, wasabi (horseradish paste), miso (fermented soybean paste), umeboshi vinegar, sea vegetable, shiitake mushroom, toasted sesame oil	sauté garlic, ginger, and scallion in peanut oil as a base for any stir-fry; add veggies and deglaze with tamari and mirin; finish with toasted sesame oil
Chinese	tamari (soy sauce), garlic, ginger, chili peppers, rice vinegar, star anise	use the same as in Japanese cooking, adding chili pepper flakes and star anise for additional seasoning
Thai	turmeric, curry powder, garlic, ginger, lime, tamarind, lemongrass, chili peppers, cilantro, Thai basil, mint, coconut milk	use the same as in Japanese cooking, adding curry powder and coconut milk, and finishing with fresh herbs
Vietnamese	tamari (soy sauce), garlic, ginger, chili peppers, lime, mint, cilantro, peanut, coconut oil	use the same as in Japanese cooking, adding fresh herbs and chopped peanuts to finish
Indonesian	tamari (soy sauce), garlic, ginger, tamarind, chili peppers, lemon, lemongrass, peanut, coconut milk	use the same as in Japanese cooking, adding sauces made with chili pepper flakes, lemongrass, lemon, coconut milk, and peanut butter
Malaysian	tamari (soy sauce), garlic, ginger, tamarind, sambal (chili paste), lemongrass, coconut milk	use the same as in Japanese cooking, adding sambal, tamarind, and coconut milk to sauces

Parsley Pistou

Similar to a pesto but without cheese or nuts, this traditional French sauce is a quick way to add fresh flavor to any pasta, veggies, or rice and bean dish. I like pouring this into a squeeze bottle and drizzling it on top of an entree or around the inside of the plate for a pretty and tasty garnish.

INGREDIENTS

» 1 large bunch of fresh flat-leafed parsley, including stems
» 1 tsp dried oregano
» 1–2 cloves garlic
» ¼ tsp sea salt
» ½ cup olive oil (approx.)
» 1–2 tsp fresh lemon juice (approx.)

Place parsley, oregano, garlic, sea salt and 1/4 cup olive oil in a food processor and pulse until parsley is roughly chopped. Add a squeeze of lemon, then turn food processor back on and drizzle in remaining oil to achieve a smooth and pourable consistency.

Pumpkinseed Pesto

Here is an affordable twist on an Italian favorite which substitutes pumpkinseeds for more expensive pine nuts. Feel free to experiment with the ingredients by using walnuts or pistachios, or herbs such as oregano, cilantro, and even mint.

INGREDIENTS

- » ½ cup raw pumpkin seeds
- » ½ cup olive oil
- » 3–4 cloves garlic
- » 1–2 tbsp mellow white miso
- » 1–2 tbsp nutritional yeast
- » ¼ cup lemon juice
- » 1 large bunch fresh basil leaves
- » 1 large bunch fresh parsley
- » ½ tsp sea salt

Process all ingredients in a food processor until creamy. If you like a "saucier" pesto, you can add a little more olive oil. Add salt and pepper to taste.

Chimichurri

This is a traditional South and Central American sauce used for marinating meat. I prefer it on top of baked tofu or pan-fried tempeh over a bed of lettuce for a spicy, refreshing salad.

INGREDIENTS

» 1 large bunch fresh Italian parsley
» ¼ cup fresh cilantro
» ½ cup olive oil
» ⅓ cup white wine vinegar
» 2 garlic cloves
» ½ tsp red pepper flakes
» ½ tsp ground cumin
» ½ tsp sea salt

Process all ingredients in a food processor until a thick sauce is created, leaving some texture. Add salt and pepper to taste.

Sofrito

This sauce is used in cooking throughout the Caribbean, and especially in Puerto Rico and the Dominican Republic. It's a fragrant blend of herbs used as the foundation of dishes such as soups, stews, or rice and beans. I love it served over tostadas.

INGREDIENTS

» 1 medium green bell pepper, seeded and diced
» 2 scallions, diced
» 2 cloves garlic, minced
» 2 tbsp jalapeno pepper, diced
» 1 bunch fresh cilantro
» ½ tsp sea salt

Process all ingredients in a food processor until a thick sauce is created, leaving some texture. Add salt and pepper to taste.

Chermoula

> This is a fresh and a pungent Moroccan herb sauce traditionally served with grilled fish. I like it on grilled tofu or tossed with roasted cauliflower and broccoli.

INGREDIENTS

- » 2 cups cilantro (2 large bunches)
- » 1 cup flat Italian parsley (1 large bunch)
- » 2–3 garlic cloves
- » ½ tsp sea salt (to taste)
- » 2 tsp ground cumin
- » 1 tsp paprika
- » ½ tsp ground coriander
- » ⅛ tsp cayenne pepper
- » ⅓ cup extra virgin olive oil
- » juice of 1 freshly squeezed lemon (about ¼ cup)

This sauce is traditionally made by mashing all of the ingredients together with a mortar and pestle, but a food processor will work just fine! Pulse together all of the ingredients to make a thick paste. Season with sea salt.

Crimini Mushroom Gravy

> This is my go-to ThanksLiving gravy recipe served over baked tofu, holiday loaf, or any plant-based meat.

INGREDIENTS

- » 1–2 tbsp olive oil
- » 8 oz. mushrooms, sliced
- » 1 clove garlic
- » 2 tbsp cornstarch
- » 3 tbsp tamari
- » 1 ½ cups water
- » 2 tbsp tahini

In a medium sauce pot, sauté mushrooms and garlic in olive oil until soft and beginning to brown, about 5 to 10 minutes. Combine cornstarch, tamari and water in a cup. Add to pot and heat until sauce thickens. Remove from heat and gradually whisk in tahini until smooth and creamy.

Harissa Sauce

Harissa is the spicy flavor foundation of Tunisian cooking. This sauce pairs well with rice and bean dishes and can even be tossed with pasta, stirred into soup, or used as a salad dressing.

INGREDIENTS

» 12 oz. jar of roasted red peppers, drained
» ¼ tsp garlic powder
» ¼ tsp cumin
» ¼ tsp coriander
» ½ tsp smoked paprika
» ⅛ tsp cayenne pepper
» ½ tsp sea salt
» 1 tbsp olive oil
» 1 tsp apple cider vinegar
» 1–2 tbsp water (as needed)

Puree ingredients in a high-speed blender until thick sauce forms, adding water if necessary.

Dijon Agave Dressing

This glaze can be drizzled over baked tofu, pan-fried tempeh, or fresh steamed veggies.

INGREDIENTS

» 2 tbsp olive oil
» 1 tbsp Dijon mustard
» 1 tsp agave syrup
» ¼ tsp sea salt

Stir together all ingredients to create a smooth sauce.

Avocado Aioli

I love putting this sauce in a squeeze bottle and drizzling it over tostadas or enchiladas. It's also delicious as a dressing for a salad.

INGREDIENTS

- » 1 avocado, pitted and peeled
- » 2 tbsp rice vinegar
- » 1 fresh organic orange, peeled and pith removed
- » 2 tbsp lime juice (juice of 2 limes)
- » ½ tsp sea salt
- » 2 tbsp agave syrup
- » 1 clove garlic
- » ⅓ cup water (approximately)

Combine all of the above ingredients in a food processor or high speed blender. Gradually add water until a smooth and creamy consistency is achieved. The texture should be thinner than guacamole, yet not too watery.

Vegan Sour Cream

This is an easy substitute if you want to eliminate excess fat from dishes that call for vegan mayonnaise.

INGREDIENTS

» ½ cup silken tofu
» 1 tsp apple cider vinegar
» 1 tsp lemon juice
» 1 tsp Dijon mustard
» ¼ tsp sea salt

Puree all of the ingredients in a blender until smooth. Alternatively, you can soak ½ cup raw cashews in water for an hour, drain, and rinse, then blend with ¼ fresh water in place of the tofu for a raw cashew mayo.

Cashew Ranch

> Serve this as a dipping sauce with Buffalo Tofu and veggies. For those with nut allergies, substitute silken tofu for the cashews.

INGREDIENTS

- » ½ cup raw cashews
- » ½ tsp garlic powder
- » 1 tsp apple cider vinegar
- » 1 tsp lemon juice
- » 1 tsp Dijon mustard
- » a few dashes of Tabasco sauce
- » ¼ tsp sea salt
- » ¼ cup water
- » 1 tbsp finely chopped fresh dill (or 1 tsp dried)

Puree all of the ingredients except dill in a blender until smooth. Pour dressing into a mason jar (or bowl) and add dill. Cover and shake till combined.

Maple Chipotle Cashew Crema

There's an addictive balance in this sauce. Just when you think it's sweet, you get a kick of smoky spice which makes you crave more sweet. A little goes a long way, so serve it on the inside perimeter of the plate with Pecan Crusted Tempeh.

INGREDIENTS

» 1 cup raw cashews (soaked at least 1 hour, drained, and rinsed)
» 1–2 tsp smoked paprika powder
» ¼ tsp chipotle chili powder
» ½ tsp apple cider vinegar
» 1 tbsp lemon juice
» 1 tbsp maple syrup
» 1 tsp sea salt
» ½ cup water

Blend all ingredients in a high-speed blender, gradually adding water to achieve a smooth consistency. Pour into squeeze bottle.

Horseradish Dijon Crema

> You'll enjoy this poured over baked tofu, dolloped on a Buckwheat Galette, or as a sandwich spread with pan-fried tempeh, tomato, lettuce, and Shiitake Bacon. For those with nut allergies, substitute silken tofu for the cashews.

INGREDIENTS

» ½ cup raw cashews (soaked in water at least one hour, drained and rinsed)
» 1–2 tbsp nutritional yeast
» approx. ½ cup water
» 1 clove minced garlic
» 1–2 tbsp horseradish
» 2 tsp Dijon mustard
» 1 tsp fresh lemon juice
» ½ tsp sea salt
» fresh black pepper

Place soaked cashews, nutritional yeast, garlic and about ¼ cup water in blender and puree, gradually adding enough water to achieve a thick, creamy consistency. Pour into small bowl and combine with mustard, lemon juice, and horseradish. Season with salt and pepper.

Tartar Sauce

> Serve this sauce drizzled over Baked Stuffed Filet of
> Tofu for an authentic taste of the sea.

INGREDIENTS

- » ½ cup cashews, soaked, drained and rinsed
- » 1 tbsp lemon juice
- » ¼ cup water, approximately
- » ½ tsp garlic powder
- » ½ tsp Dijon mustard
- » ½ tsp sea salt
- » ¼ cup fresh dill, minced
- » 2 tsp capers
- » 1 tbsp relish or chopped pickle

Place cashews in blender with lemon juice, garlic powder, mustard, sea salt, and enough water to form a thick, smooth cream. Pour into bowl and stir in remaining ingredients. Mixture should have a slightly chunky texture.

Sundried Tomato Tapanade

This is a versatile sauce that can be used as a dip, spread on toasted baguette or a sandwich, slathered on baked tofu or tempeh, stirred into sauces or soups, or tossed with pasta.

INGREDIENTS

» ¼ cup walnuts
» 8 sundried tomatoes
» ½ cup kalamata olives
» 2 cloves garlic, minced
» 3 tbsp chopped fresh parsley
» ¼ cup chopped fresh basil
» Sea salt to taste
» 2 tbsp extra virgin olive oil

In a food processor, pulse walnuts until roughly chopped. Add remaining ingredients and pulse 5 to 6 times until coarsely chopped, then scrape down the sides with a spatula. Gradually add olive oil and blend to form a thick paste, leaving some texture.

Maple Pumpkin Sauce

This is a simple, sweet and spicy dessert sauce that's pretty when drizzled from a squeeze bottle onto the plate for a festive flare. I like it with Dirty Blondies or Chocolate Kahlua Brownies.

INGREDIENTS

» 3 tbsp canned pumpkin puree
» 3 tbsp maple syrup
» ⅛ tsp sea salt
» ⅛ tsp cinnamon
» 1–2 tbsp water

Place all of the above ingredients into a squeeze bottle, shaking together vigorously until smooth, adding water as necessary.

Berry Sauce

> Spread a pool of this sauce on the plate before adding your dessert or place it in a squeeze bottle for some fun drizzling. Pairs well with chocolate dessert of any kind, as a sauce for pancakes, or on top of vanilla ice cream.

INGREDIENTS

» 1 10 oz. jar of seedless preserves (raspberry, blueberry, strawberry, or even apricot)
» 1 tbsp maple syrup
» 1 tbsp water

Blend all of the above ingredients together in a high-speed blender until smooth and slightly foamy. Pour into squeeze bottle and squeeze sauce onto dessert.

Chocolate Ganache

This is a rich sauce that is delicious on brownies or ice-cream or for dipped strawberries. It firms up when cool, so be sure to plan in advance when using it.

INGREDIENTS

» 1 tbsp coconut oil
» 8 oz. dark chocolate, chopped (use a solid bar rather than chocolate chips)

Melt coconut oil in a sauce pot on low heat. Add chopped chocolate and stir together until melted, being careful not to overheat.

Desserts

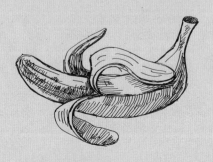

— Desserts —
(with gluten-free modifications)

Family favorites can easily be veganized simply by substituting plant-based milk for dairy, vegan margarine or coconut oil for butter, and any of the egg substitutes listed in the previous chapter. If a recipe calls for sugar, use vegan sugar that isn't filtered with bone char.; for honey, substitute agave or maple syrup. Whether it's cookies or cake, muffins or brownies, you're family won't notice the difference. What follows are a few of my favorites that have become new family traditions.

Kahlua Brownies with Chocolate Ganache
(serves 9)

These are moist and dense brownies made even richer when topped with a coating of Chocolate Ganache. Feel free to vary this recipe by sprinkling with chopped walnuts or shredded coconut.

INGREDIENTS

» ½ cup quick oats
» ½ cup organic sugar
» 1 tsp baking powder
» ¼ tsp sea salt
» ½ cup cocoa powder
» 1 15 oz. can black beans, drained and rinsed
» 3 tbsp Kahlua
» 3 tbsp coconut oil, melted
» ¼ cup applesauce
» ¼ cup maple syrup or agave syrup
» 2 tsp pure vanilla extract

Preheat oven to 350°F. Lightly oil an 8 × 8 baking pan. Combine ingredients in a food processor and blend for several minutes until batter is smooth, scraping down sides as needed. Pour batter into the pan. Bake for 30 to 40 minutes or until the top is dry and edges are starting to pull away from the sides. Let cool for 30 minutes in the pan, then top with Chocolate Ganache (see p. 222). Refrigerate at least an hour to stiffen before serving. Carefully slice into 9 or 12 squares, and gently remove with a spatula.

Dirty Blondies
(serves 9)

> This dessert is so moist and decadent you'd never know the secret ingredient is beans. Eat them for a guilt-free dessert or a grab-and-go snack.

INGREDIENTS

» ½ cup quick oats
» ¾ cup organic brown sugar
» 1 tsp baking powder
» ¼ tsp salt
» 1 15 oz. cans white beans, drained and rinsed
» ¼ cup applesauce
» 2 tbsp coconut oil
» 1 tsp pure vanilla extract
» ½ cup chocolate chips (Enjoy Life mini chips)
» ⅓ cup chopped pecans
» ⅓ cup shredded unsweetened coconut

Preheat oven to 350°F. Blend all of the ingredients except the chocolate chips, pecans, and coconut in a large food processor until a smooth batter forms. Pulse all but 2 tbsp each of chocolate chips, pecans, and coconut into batter, then spread into an oiled 8 × 8 pan. Sprinkle reserved ingredients evenly over the top. Bake for around 35 to 45 minutes, or until top is firm and sides are beginning to brown and pull away from the pan. Let cool at least 10 minutes, then gently cut into squares and remove from the pan. Best after refrigerated several hours or overnight.

Variations: Alternatively, you can double the recipe and pour the batter into an oiled 10-inch tart pan to make an elegant presentation. In the fall I like to substitute pumpkin puree for the applesauce and add ½ tsp cinnamon, ⅛ tsp of allspice, and ⅛ tsp powdered ginger.

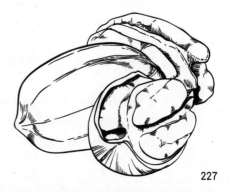

Lemon Coconut Bundt Cake with Coconut Glaze

(serves 8 to 10)

> I love this dessert in the spring when violets and pansies are in bloom for a beautiful edible flower garnish. Alternatively, in the summer I garnish this cake with plump local blueberries which contrast nicely with the tart lemon. A drizzle of Berry Coulis on the plate adds to the flavor explosion.

CAKE INGREDIENTS

» 3 ⅓ cups all purpose flour (or substitute 3 cups Bob's Redmill gluten-free flour, ⅓ cup brown rice flour, and 1 tsp xanthan gum)
» 2 tsp baking powder
» 1 tsp baking soda
» ½ tsp sea salt
» 1 ½ cups unsweetened coconut milk from carton (not canned)
» ¼ cup fresh lemon juice
» 1 ¾ cups organic cane sugar
» ½ cup unsweetened applesauce
» ½ cup coconut oil, melted
» 2 tsp lemon zest
» 1 ½ tsp pure vanilla extract
» 1 ½ tsp lemon extract

COCONUT GLAZE INGREDIENTS

» 1 ½ cups organic powdered sugar
» 1–2 Tbsp coconut milk
» ½ tsp pure vanilla extract

Preheat oven to 350 °F. Oil bundt cake pan then set aside. In large mixing bowl, sift together dry ingredients. In separate bowl, mix together coconut milk and lemon juice, and let sit until curdled. Add sugar, applesauce, oil, lemon zest, vanilla and lemon extract. Pour over flour mixture and stir to combine. Pour batter into prepared bundt cake pan. Bake for 40 to 45 minutes or until toothpick inserted in cake comes out clean. Allow to cool in pan for 10 minutes before removing from pan. Continue to cool on cooling rack.

Blueberry Almond Cobbler
(serves 4 to 6)

> Think of a cobbler like a giant deconstructed muffin. The batter goes in first, then as if you forgot to add the berries, you just dump them over the top. They cook and spread and melt together into a nice yummy mess with the moist cake batter underneath. Use fresh or frozen blueberries for this recipe, or substitute any wild foraged berry depending on the season.

INGREDIENTS

- » 1 ¼ cups all purpose flour (or substitute 1 cup gluten-free flour, ¼ cup rice flour, plus ½ tsp xanthan gum)
- » ½ cup sugar
- » ¼ tsp sea salt
- » 1 ½ tsp baking powder
- » ¾ cup almond milk
- » ¼ tsp almond extract
- » ⅓ cup vegan margarine, melted
- » 2 cups blueberries
- » ⅓ cup slivered almonds
- » ⅓ cup organic sugar
- » ½ tsp cinnamon
- » 1 tsp vanilla extract

Preheat oven to 350°F. In a large mixing bowl, stir together flour, sugar, salt, and baking powder. Stir in milk, almond extract, and melted margarine till combined. Pour batter into an oiled 8-inch square baking pan. In a separate mixing bowl, toss blueberries, almonds, sugar, cinnamon, and vanilla extract together, then sprinkle mixture evenly over batter. Bake for 55 to 60 minutes or until firm to the touch and top is lightly browned.

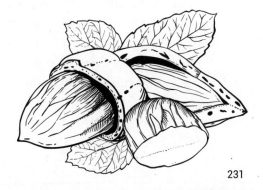

Apple Crisp

(serves 4 to 6)

> This is an easy recipe perfect for enjoying after a day of picking apples and raking leaves.

FILLING INGREDIENTS

» 6 cups sweet apples, cored and diced (about 5 to 6 apples)
» 2 tsp lemon juice
» 1 tbsp maple syrup
» 1 tsp vanilla
» ½ tsp cinnamon

TOPPING INGREDIENTS

» ½ cup almonds, ground into a fine meal
» ½ cup all-purpose flour (or substitute gluten-free flour)
» 1 tsp cinnamon
» ½ cup organic brown sugar
» ⅓ cup coconut oil, melted
» 2 tbsp maple syrup

Preheat oven to 375 °F. Place apples in an oiled 8 × 8" pan. Mix with lemon juice, maple syrup, vanilla, and cinnamon. In a large bowl, mix together ground almonds, buckwheat flour, cinnamon, sugar, and melted coconut oil until it clumps together. Sprinkle topping over apple mixture, then drizzle with maple syrup. Cover with aluminum foil and bake for 30 to 40 minutes, then uncover and bake another 15 to 20 minutes, or until bubbly and beginning to brown.

Grandma's Lithuanian Apple Cake

(serves 10 to 12)

> This dessert is like a childhood memory for me. My grandmother never wrote her recipe down, but I remember her coring and cutting apple after apple after apple from the big tree in her back yard. I played with this until I got just the right consistency. It's super moist and dense. You'll think there are too many apples, but once they cook down it'll all turn out ok.

INGREDIENTS

» 1 ½ cups all-purpose gluten-free flour
» ½ cup brown rice flour
» ½ tsp xanthan gum
» 1 tsp baking soda
» 1 tsp cinnamon
» 1 tsp sea salt
» 1 ½ cups Sucanat (unrefined cane syrup)
» 3 tbsp ground flax seeds, plus 1/3 cup water
» ¼ cup coconut oil, melted
» ¼ cup applesauce
» ½ cup apple cider
» 1 tsp vanilla
» 3 cups peeled and sliced apples
» ½ cup chopped walnuts

Preheat oven to 375°F. In a large mixing bowl, sift together flour, xanthan gum, baking soda, cinnamon and salt. In a separate bowl, mix together Sucanat, flax seed mixture, oil, cider and vanilla. Combine wet and dry ingredients and stir until smooth. Stir in apples and walnuts. Spread batter into oiled 9 × 13 pan and bake 40 to 50 minutes, or until edges are lightly browned and toothpick comes out clean. Let cook, then top with powdered sugar if desired.

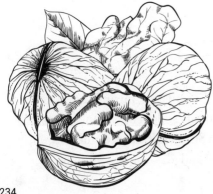

Double Chocolate Cupcakes
(makes 1 dozen)

> This is my "go to" chocolate cake recipe. It's decadent and versatile and can be topped with chopped walnuts, fresh berries, or crushed peppermint stick depending on the occasion.

CUPCAKE INGREDIENTS

» 1 ½ cups all-purpose gluten-free flour
» 1 cup vegan sugar
» 4 tbsp cocoa powder
» ½ tsp xanthan gum
» 1 tsp baking soda
» ½ tsp sea salt
» 1 ¼ cups water
» ¼ cup applesauce
» ¼ cup canola oil
» 1 tbsp vinegar
» 1 tsp vanilla

Preheat oven to 350°F. Sift dry ingredients together in a large bowl. In a separate bowl, combine wet ingredients. Pour wet ingredients into dry ingredients and stir until there are no lumps. Pour batter into a muffin tin lined with muffin cups. Bake for 12 to 18 minutes. Gently remove from muffin tin and let cool on a wire rack before frosting.

CHOCOLATE FROSTING INGREDIENTS

» ¼ cup vegan margarine
» ⅓ cup cocoa powder
» 1 ½ cups confectioners sugar
» 3 tbsp almond milk, approximately
» ½ tsp vanilla extract

Melt the margarine, then mix together in a bowl with cocoa powder. Alternately stir in sugar and almond milk to achieve a smooth consistency. Stir in vanilla. Frosting can be spread on cupcakes or spooned into a pastry bag for piping.

Snowball Cookies

(makes 3 dozen)

> These were a treat growing up when my mom would make containers of Christmas cookies to give away. She called them "Butterballs," but the vegan version is made without butter and I associate them with the winter holidays. Who wouldn't want to get into a snowball fight with these?

INGREDIENTS

- » 1 cup pecans
- » 1 cup all purpose gluten free flour
- » ¾ cup sorghum flour
- » ¼ tsp xanthan gum
- » ¼ tsp sea salt
- » ¾ cup vegan margarine
- » ½ cup confectioner's sugar, plus ½ cup for dusting
- » 1 tbsp maple syrup
- » ½ tsp vanilla extract

Preheat oven to 325°F. In a food processor, finely chop pecans to a flour-like consistency. Mix together in a bowl with flour, xanthan gum, and sea salt. Place margarine, sugar, maple syrup and vanilla in food processor and cream together until smooth. Add flour mixture and pulse together until just combined. Scoop out batter with a tbsp and roll into 1-inch balls. Place on engrossed baking sheet and bake for 8 to 10 minutes, or until bottoms are golden brown. Meanwhile, put about ½ cup of confectioner's sugar into a bowl. When cookies are done and still warm, very gently remove from pan and coat each individually with sugar. Be careful when handling as these are very delicate, but they will firm up as the sugar adheres and the cookie cools.

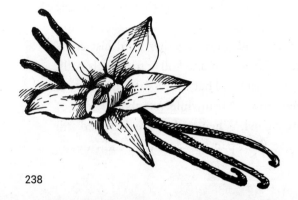

Carrot Cake with Cream Cheese Frosting
(serves 8 to 10)

> This is my mom's signature dessert that I ask for every birthday. It's dense and decadent and people will never suspect it's vegan.

CAKE INGREDIENTS

» 2 cups unsifted all-purpose flour (or 2 cups gluten-free flour plus ½ tsp xanthan gum)
» 2 tsp baking soda
» 1 tsp cinnamon
» ½ tsp ground ginger
» ½ tsp sea salt
» 3 tbsp ground flax seed plus ⅓ cup water
» 1 ¼ cups sugar
» ¾ cup canola oil
» 8 oz. can crushed pineapple, undrained
» 2 cups shredded carrots
» ¾ cup chopped walnuts

Grease and flour two 9-inch round pans. In a bowl, stir together dry ingredients, then set aside. In a large bowl, whisk together flax seed mixture, sugar, oil, and pineapple until well mixed. Gradually stir in flour mixture until well mixed. Gently str in carrots and walnuts and mix until blended together. Pour into prepared cake pans and bake for 30 to 35 minutes, or until toothpick inserted in center comes out clean. Cool in pans for 10 minutes, then turn onto rack to cool completely.

FROSTING INGREDIENTS

- » 6 oz. vegan cream cheese
- » 3 cups confectioners sugar
- » 2 tbsp vegan margarine
- » 1 tsp vanilla

Cream ingredients together in a food processor or mixer until smooth and fluffy. Frost both layers of cake with frosting to make a double layer cake. Garnish with chopped walnuts or shredded coconut (optional).

Strawberry Shortcake

(makes 2 dozen)

> This is a vegan twist on a classic recipe. I use muffin tins to make the shortcake, then slice them in half to layer with strawberries and Coconut Whip Cream. Alternatively, it can be layered in pretty wine glasses with berries and cream for an elegant parfait. It's the perfect dessert for summer picnics when local berries are in season.

INGREDIENTS

- » 2 cups all-purpose flour (or substitute all-purpose gluten-free flour plus ¼ tsp xanthan gum)
- » 2 tsp baking powder
- » ½ tsp baking soda
- » ½ tsp sea salt
- » 1 cup organic sugar
- » 1 ½ cups almond milk mixed with 1 tbsp apple cider vinegar
- » ½ cup canola oil
- » 1 ¼ tsp vanilla extract
- » 10 oz. fresh strawberries, tops removed and sliced

Preheat oven to 350°F. Prepare muffin tins with 24 paper liners. Sift together dry ingredients in a large bowl. Add wet ingredients and whisk until there are no lumps. Fill each muffin cup about ¾ full. Bake 15 to 20 minutes, or until light and springy and a toothpick comes out clean. Cool shortcakes and carefully remove from paper liner before serving topped with fresh strawberries and Coconut Whip Cream (see p. 244).

Apple Cinnamon Bread Pudding with Maple Pecan Glaze

(serves 8 to 12)

> This was a big hit at my New Year's Day Vegan Brunch. It's kinda like French toast, but in casserole form, so it serves a crowd and you don't need to stand in front of a hot skillet flipping toast all afternoon. It's delicious eaten warm straight out of the oven or chilled after it gets more pudding-like.

BREAD PUDDING INGREDIENTS

» 3 cups almond milk
» ½ cup sugar
» 1 tsp vanilla
» 1 tbsp corn starch
» ¼ tsp sea salt
» 9–10 slices of bread cut into cubes (about 4 cups)
» 4 apples, cored, peeled, and diced
» ½ cup sugar mixed with ½ tsp cinnamon (sprinkle over top)

Preheat oven to 375°F. Whisk together almond milk, sugar, vanilla, corn starch and sea salt in a large bowl. Submerge cubed bread and let sit for a half an hour to soak up the liquid. Toss with apples, then pour into oiled 9 × 13 pan. Sprinkle with sugar and cinnamon mixture, then cover with foil and bake for 35 to 45 minutes, or until bread is puffed and liquid is bubbly. Remove foil and bake another 15 to 20 minutes to brown top. Remove from oven and prepare Maple Pecan Glaze.

MAPLE PECAN GLAZE INGREDIENTS

» ½ cup chopped pecans
» 2 tbsp vegan margarine
» ¼ cup maple syrup
» pinch of sea salt

Just before serving the bread pudding, heat pecans, margarine and maple syrup in a pan on medium heat until bubbly. Pour over the top of pudding and serve while warm.

Coconut Whip Cream

This recipe is modified from the brilliant Minimalist Baker, who discovered that canned coconut milk is perfect for whipping. You'll want to serve this with fresh berries, on top of pancakes, or any vegan dessert to make it extra decadent. I always keep a couple cans of coconut milk in my refrigerator so I can whip this up at a moment's notice.

INGREDIENTS

» 1 14 oz. can of full fat coconut milk that has been chilled overnight
» ½ cup confectioners sugar
» ½ tsp vanilla extract

Open the chilled can of coconut milk and carefully remove only the hard, thickened cream, leaving the liquid behind. Place cream in food processor and whip till smooth. Add vanilla and powdered sugar and mix for about a minute, or until creamy and no lumps remain. You can use this immediately for a soft cream, or refrigerate it several hours to firm up. Stir together before dolloping liberally on top of your favorite dessert.

Chocolate Black Bean Truffles
(makes 3 dozen)

> I'm not sure who came up with the idea of putting black beans in truffles first, but it was pure genius. Who would guess the decadence of a chocolate truffle was hiding the health benefits of beans? This recipe is modified from one I found on the Soul Fire Farm website. They're a fabulous organization committed to ending racism and injustice in the food system, so check them out while snacking on these treats!

INGREDIENTS

- » 3 tbsp coconut oil
- » ½ cup brown sugar
- » 1 15 oz. can black beans, drained and rinsed
- » ½ cup dried cranberries
- » ¼ cup unsweetened cocoa powder
- » 1 tsp vanilla
- » ⅛ tsp sea salt
- » ½ cup coco powder (for dredging)
- » ½ cup shredded coconut (for dredging)

In a small skillet, heat coconut oil and brown sugar on low heat until melted. Next, pulse together black beans and dried cranberries in a food processor fitted with the metal blade. Add oil and sugar mixture and remaining ingredients, then blend until smooth. Using a spatula, pour batter into a bowl and spread out so that it's about an inch thick. Place in the refrigerator for about an hour to firm up. Using a melon baller or a tbsp, soup out the truffle mixture and roll into balls a little bit larger than a marble. After the truffles have been rolled, dredge half in the cocoa powder and half in the shredded coconut, pressing to stick. Place in a container and refrigerate prior to serving.

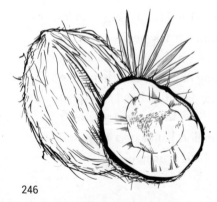

RAW Chocomole

(serves 2 to 4)

Ever open a soft, ripe avocado only to find it's nearly brown inside? No worries! Make Chocomole instead of guacamole! This pudding needs no cooking and takes just minutes to make and enjoy.

INGREDIENTS

- » 2 ripe avocados, peeled, pitted, and cubed
- » ½ cup agave syrup
- » 1 tsp vanilla
- » ¼ cup unrefined coconut oil, melted
- » ½ cup unsweetened cocoa powder
- » pinch of sea salt
- » ½ cup water (approx.)

In a food processor, puree avocados, agave, and vanilla until smooth. Add coconut oil, cocoa powder, and sea salt and puree until creamy, adding water if necessary. Refrigerate 1 hour before serving and top with sliced bananas, fresh berries or chopped walnuts and a dollop of coconut whip.

RAW Fruit Tart with Date Nut Crust

(serves 6 to 8)

> If you're looking for a healthy dessert recipe that will wow everyone at a party, this is the one to bring. It's as beautiful as it is delicious, and it's loaded with the health benefits of antioxidants from the fresh fruit. Let your kids have fun by layering fruit in their own creative patterns.

CRUST INGREDIENTS

» 1 cup walnuts (soaked 1 hour, drained, and rinsed)
» 1 cup pecans (soaked 1 hour, drained, and rinsed)
» ½ cup dried coconut
» 10 Medjool dates, pitted
» 1 tsp cinnamon
» pinch of sea salt

Coarsely chop walnuts and pecans in a food processor. Then add dates, coconut, cinnamon and sea salt, and blend until it begins to stick together. Press into an 8-inch tart pan and refrigerate while preparing the fruit topping.

TOPPING INGREDIENTS

» 2 bananas, sliced into ¼-inch rounds
» 1 kiwi, sliced into ½-inch half moons
» 8 oz. strawberries, sliced
» 8 oz. blueberries
» 1–2 tbsp agave syrup (optional)

Place bananas evenly in a layer around bottom of crust. Top with sliced kiwi, then strawberry in an overlapping spiral. Place blueberries in the center, then drizzle top with agave syrup.

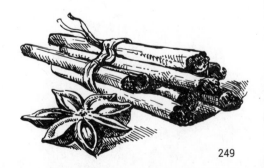

Cooking Conversions

Volume Conversions: Normally used for liquids only	
Customary quantity	**Metric equivalent**
1 teaspoon	5 mL
1 tablespoon or ½ fluid ounce	15 mL
1 fluid ounce or ⅛ cup	30 mL
¼ cup or 2 fluid ounces	60 mL
⅓ cup	80 mL
½ cup or 4 fluid ounces	120 mL
⅔ cup	160 mL
¾ cup or 6 fluid ounces	180 mL
1 cup or 8 fluid ounces or half a pint	240 mL
1 ½ cups or 12 fluid ounces	350 mL
2 cups or 1 pint or 16 fluid ounces	475 mL
3 cups or 1 ½ pints	700 mL
4 cups or 2 pints or 1 quart	950 mL
4 quarts or 1 gallon	3.8 L

Note: In cases where higher precision is not justified, it may be convenient to round these conversions off as follows:

1 cup = 250 mL
1 pint = 500 mL
1 quart = 1 L
1 gallon = 4 L

Weight Conversions	
Customary quantity	**Metric equivalent**
1 ounce	28 g
4 ounces or ¼ pound	113 g
⅓ pound	150 g
8 ounces or ½ pound	230 g
⅔ pound	300 g
12 ounces or ¾ pound	340 g
1 pound or 16 ounces	450 g
2 pounds	900 g

Cooking Times		
°F	**°C**	**Gas mark**
275°F	140°C	gas mark 1
300°F	150°C	gas mark 2
325°F	165°C	gas mark 3
350°F	180°C	gas mark 4
375°F	190°C	gas mark 5
400°F	200°C	gas mark 6
425°F	220°C	gas mark 7
450°F	230°C	gas mark 9
475°F	240°C	gas mark 10

Weights of common ingredients in grams

Ingredient	1 cup	¾ cup	⅔ cup	½ cup	⅓ cup	¼ cup	2 Tbsp
Flour, all purpose (wheat)	120 g	90 g	80 g	60 g	40 g	30 g	15 g
Flour, well sifted all purpose (wheat)	110 g	80 g	70 g	55 g	35 g	27 g	13 g
Sugar, granulated cane	200 g	150 g	130 g	100 g	65 g	50 g	25 g
Confectioner's sugar (cane)	100 g	75 g	70 g	50 g	35 g	25 g	13 g
Brown sugar, packed firmly (but not too firmly)	180 g	135 g	120 g	90 g	60 g	45 g	23 g
Corn meal	160 g	120 g	100 g	80 g	50 g	40 g	20 g
Corn starch	120 g	90 g	80 g	60 g	40 g	30 g	15 g
Rice, uncooked	190 g	140 g	125 g	95 g	65 g	48 g	24 g
Macaroni, uncooked	140 g	100 g	90 g	70 g	45 g	35 g	17 g
Couscous, uncooked	180 g	135 g	120 g	90 g	60 g	45 g	22 g
Oats, uncooked quick	90 g	65 g	60 g	45 g	30 g	22 g	11 g
Table salt	300 g	230 g	200 g	150 g	100 g	75 g	40 g
Vegan Butter	240 g	180 g	160 g	120 g	80 g	60 g	30 g
Vegetable shortening	190 g	140 g	125 g	95 g	65 g	48 g	24 g
Chopped fruits and vegetables	150 g	110 g	100 g	75 g	50 g	40 g	20 g
Nuts, chopped	150 g	110 g	100 g	75 g	50 g	40 g	20 g
Nuts, ground	120 g	90 g	80 g	60 g	40 g	30 g	15 g
Bread crumbs, fresh, loosely packed	60 g	45 g	40 g	30 g	20 g	15 g	8 g
Bread crumbs, dry	150 g	110 g	100 g	75 g	50 g	40 g	20 g
Vegan cheese, grated	90 g	65 g	60 g	45 g	30 g	22 g	11 g

Recipe Index

BREAKFAST
- Breakfast Tostadas 108
- Buckwheat Galette with Spinach, Mushroom, and Fennel Seed 119
- Cranberry Muffins with Toasted Coconut Almond Streusel 112
- Loaded Oatmeal 114
- Old-Fashioned Banana Bread 117
- Perfect Pancakes 110
- Pina Colada Congee 116
- RAW Overnight Banana Berry Chia Pudding 123
- Smoked Paprika Home-fried Potatoes 109
- Southwestern Tofu Scramble 107
- Tofu Florentine Quiche 121

LUNCH
Salads
- Greek Lentil and Brown Rice Salad with Lemon and Olives 137
- Mediterranean Quinoa Salad 129
  Shaved Brussels Sprout Salad 135
- Tri-Color Slaw 128
- Warm Walnut, Carrot, Snow Pea, and Brown Rice Salad 131
- World Peas Salad 133

Soups
- Berbere Spiced Lentils with Lemon and Spinach 141
- Butternut Squash Bisque 145
- Curried Red Lentil Soup 139
- Garden Veggie Soup 143
- Rootsy Chowder.. 146

Sandwiches and Wraps
- Barbecue Jackfruit Sliders 148
- Eggless Egg Salad 152

- Fire Breathing Dragon Salad 153
- Mediterranean Tofu 159
- Mock Chicken Salad 151
- Portobello Pate 158
- Tempeh Tartare on Avocado Toast 154
- Unfried Beans 156

DINNER
Entrees
- Baked Stuffed Filet of Tofu 175
- Baked Stuffed Zucchini Romesco............................... 180
- Buffalo Tofu 174
- Butternut Squash "Steaks" with Walnut Mushroom Cream 178
- Lasagna with Summer Squash 172
- Moroccan Chickpea Tagine 183
- Pan-seared Tempeh with Fig and Balsamic Reduction Sauce 176
- Pecan Crusted Tempeh 163
- Roasted Eggplant and Tofu Stacks with Fire Roasted Tomato Marinara 169
- Seared Mushroom "Scallops" with Lemon Caper Sauce 181
- Tempeh Stroganoff 165
- Walnut and Spinach Pesto Stuffed Portobello Caps.... 167

Sides
- Asian Sesame Cabbage 199
- Avocado Fries 194
- Besan Cakes 200
- Black-eyed Pea Fritters 187
- Chili Lime Corn on the Cob 193
- Garnet Yam Hash 191
- Jamaican Sautéed Black Beans, Greens, and Garnet Yam 189
- Mashed Root Vegetables 190
- Roasted Asparagus 201
- Sesame String Beans 196

- Shiitake Bacon 197
- String Bean Amandine 198
- Zucchini Fritters 185

Sauces and Flavor Bursts
- Avocado Aioli 213
- Berry Sauce 221
- Cashew Ranch 215
- Chermoula 209
- Chimichurri 207
- Chocolate Ganache 222
- Crimini Mushroom Gravy.................... 210
- Dijon Agave Dressing 212
- Harissa Sauce 211
- Horseradish Dijon Crema 217
- Maple Chipotle Cashew Crema 216
- Maple Pumpkin Sauce 220
- Parsley Pistou 205
- Pumpkinseed Pesto 206
- Sofrito 208
- Sundried Tomato Tapanade 219
- Tartar Sauce 218
- Vegan Sour Cream 214

DESSERTS (with gluten-free modifications)
- Apple Cinnamon Bread Pudding with Maple Pecan
  Glaze 242
- Apple Crisp 232
- Blueberry Almond Cobbler 230
- Carrot Cake with Cream Cheese Frosting 239
- Chocolate Black Bean Truffles 245
- Coconut Whip Cream 244
- Dirty Blondies 226
- Double Chocolate Cupcakes 235
- Grandma's Lithuanian Apple Cake 233
- Kahlua Brownies with Chocolate Ganache 225
- Lemon Coconut Bundt Cake with Coconut Glaze 228
- RAW Chocomole 247

- RAW Fruit Tart with Date Nut Crust 248
- Snowball Cookies 237
- Strawberry Shortcake 241

Appendix – Resources

Activism and Advocacy

- Adams, Carol J. *Living Among Meat Eaters: The Vegetarians' Survival Handbook.* New York: Lantern, 2009.
- Colb, Sherry F. *Mind If I Order the Cheeseburger? And Other Questions People Ask Vegans.* New York: Lantern, 2013.
- Francione, Gary L. and Anna Charlton. *Eat Like You Care: An Examination of the Morality of Eating Animals.* USA: Exempla Press, 2015.
- Grillo, Robert. *Farm to Fable: The Fictions of Our Animal-Consuming Culture.* Danvers, MA: Vegan Publishers, 2016.
- jones, pattrice. *Aftershock: Confronting Trauma in a Violent World.* New York: Lantern, 2007.
- Joy, Melanie, and John Robbins. *Why We Love Dogs, Eat Pigs, and Wear Cows: An Introduction to Carnism: The Belief System That Enables Us to Eat Some Animals and Not Others.* San Francisco: Conari Press, 2011.
- Taft, Casey T. *Motivational Methods for Vegan Advocacy: A Clinical Psychology Perspective.* Danvers, MA: Vegan Publishers, 2016.

Animal Rescue Organizations

- Best Friends Animal Society, Kanab, UT (www.bestfriends.org)
- Catskill Farm Animal Sanctuary, Saugerties, NY (www.casanctuary.org)
- Farm Sanctuary, Watkins Glen, NY (www.farmsanctuary.org)
- Maple Farm Sanctuary, Methuen, MA (www.maplefarmsanctuary.org)
- VINE Sanctuary, Springfield, VT (http://vine.bravebirds.org)
- Woodstock Farm Sanctuary, High Falls, NY (www.woodstocksanctuary.org)

Basic Vegan Information

- Food Studies Institute (www.foodstudies.org)
- Veg Web (www.vegweb.com/vegan101)
- The Vegan Society (www.vegansociety.com)

- Vegetarian Resource Group (www.vrg.org/nutshell/vegan. htm)
- Physicians Committee for Responsible Medicine (www. pcrm.org/health/diets)

Documentaries
- *Blackfish*
- *The Cove*
- *Cowspiracy*
- *Earthlings*
- *Forks Over Knives*
- *The Ghosts in Our Machine*
- *Peaceable Kingdom*
- *Plant Pure Nation*
- *Speciesism: The Movie*
- *Tyke: Elephant Outlaw*
- *Unlocking the Cage*
- *Vegucated*
- *What the Health*

Humane Education
- The Compassionate Living Project (www.compassionate livingproject.org)
- Institute for Humane Education (www.humaneeducation. org)
- Humane Education Advocates Reaching Teachers (www. teachhumane.org/heart)

Non-Profit Organizations
- A Well-fed World (www.awfw.org)
- American Vegan Society (www.americanvegan.org)
- Animal Legal Defense Fund (www.aldf.org)
- Coalition for Healthy School Food (www.healthyschoolfood. org)
- FARM USA (www.farmusa.org)
- Food Empowerment Project (www.foodispower.org)
- Food For Life Global (www.ffl.org)
- Food Not Bombs (http://www.foodnotbombs.net/new_site)

- Non-Human Rights Project (www.nonhumanrightsproject. org)
- North American Vegetarian Society (www.navs-online.org)
- Physicians Committee for Responsible Medicine (www. pcrm.org)
- Tribe of Heart (www.tribeofheart.org)
- Vegan Outreach (www.veganoutreach.org)

Vegan Nutrition
- Dr. Michael Greger (www.nutritionfacts.org)
- Ginny Kisch Messina (www.theveganrd.com)
- Brenda Davis (www.brendadavisrd.com)
- Julieanna Hever (www.plantbaseddietician.com)
- Jack Norris (www.jacknorrisrd.com)

Vegan Products and Brands
- Beyond Meat (www.beyondmeat.com) – Beyond Burger, Beast Burger, beefless crumbles and strips
- Bionaturae (www.bionaturae.com) – tomato paste
- Brad's Organic (www.bradsorganic.com) – nut butters, tahini
- The Bridge (www.bridgetofu.com) – tofu
- Daiya (http://us.daiyafoods.com) – vegan cheese and spreads
- Earth Balance (www.earthbalancenatural.com) – vegan margarine, spreads, mayo
- Eden Organic (www.edenfoods.com) – canned beans
- Field Roast (www.fieldroast.com) – vegan meats, Chao cheese
- Follow Your Heart (www.followyourheart.com) – Vegenaise vegan mayonnaise, The Vegan Egg, nondairy cheese, yogurt
- Hampton Creek (www.hamptoncreek.com) – Just Mayo vegan mayonnaise, salad dressing, cookie dough, cookies
- Kite Hill (www.kite-hill.com) – nut-based cheeses, cream cheese, ricotta, sour cream, and yogurt
- Lightlife (www.lightlife.com) – tempeh products
- Miyoko's Kitchen (www.miyokoskitchen.com) – nut-based cheeses and vegan butter
- Mori Nu (www.morinu.com) – silken tofu
- Muir Glen (www.muirglen.com) – fire-roasted tomatoes

- Nutiva (www.nutiva.com) – raw hemp seeds, chia seeds, coconut oil
- Pacific Foods (www.pacificfoods) – nondairy beverages
- Rice Dream (www.tastethedream.com) – nondairy beverages, frozen desserts
- San-J (www.san-j.com) – tamari
- So Delicious (www.sodeliciousdairyfree.com) – nondairy beverages and frozen desserts
- Thai Kitchen (www.thaikitchen.com) – coconut milk, rice noodles
- Tinkyada (www.tinkyada.com) – rice pasta
- Treeline Cheese (www.treelinecheese.com) – nut-based cheeses
- Turtle Island Foods "Tofurky" (www.tofurky.com) – faux meat products
- Westbrae Naturals (www.westbrae.com) – canned beans
- Wholesome Sweeteners (www.wholesomesweeteners.com) – Sucanat, organic sugar, raw agave syrup

Vegan Restaurant Guides
- Happy Cow (www.happycow.net)
- Veg Dining (www.vegdining.com)
- Veg Guide (www.vegguide.org)

Vegan Shopping
- Alternative Outfitters (www.alternativeoutfitters.com)
- Herbivore Clothing (www.herbivoreclothing.com)
- Vegan Chic (www.veganchic.com)
- Vegan Essentials (www.veganessentials.com)
- Vegan Store (www.veganstore.com)

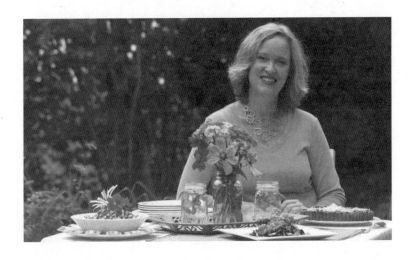

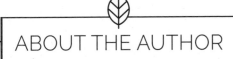

ABOUT THE AUTHOR

Mary Lawrence is a vegan wellness educator and executive chef of Connecticut's premier vegan personal chef service, Well on Wheels (www.wellonwheels.com). She offers whole foods plant-based meals prepared in clients' homes, cooking classes, corporate wellness workshops, vegan wellness jumpstarts, and private cooking and raw food lessons.

She is board member of the American Vegan Society and a frequent speaker at conferences and seminars, including the North American Vegetarian Society's annual Summerfest, the Boston Vegetarian Society, and Northeast Organic Farming Association (NOFA). She has been a guest on Our Hen House, Vegan Radio, and The Dr. Don Show. In 2007 she published her first cookbook, *Quick and Easy Vegan Cuisine*, and contributed to the Friends of Animals' cookbook, *The Best of Vegan Cooking* (2009). Her second cookbook, *Easy Peasy Vegan Eats* (2014), is a guide for people making the vegan transition. She can be followed on the blog, The Traveling Vegan Chef (http://wellonwheels. blogspot.com) and Instagram @wellonwheels.

Mary earned a certificate in plant-based nutrition from the Dr. T. Colin Campbell Foundation at eCornell University, an MA in Communication with concentration in Cultural Studies from the University of Hartford, and a BA in English from the University of Connecticut. She has been an adjunct professor at Gateway Community College in New Haven, Connecticut, for many years. She studied culinary arts at the Natural Gourmet Institute in New York City and trained in the kitchen of It's Only Natural restaurant in Middletown, Connecticut.